GOOD HOUSEKEEPING

DOCTORS' SECRETS

GOOD HOUSEKEEPING

DOCTORS' SECRETS

Fight Disease • Relieve Pain • Live a Healthy Life

with Practical Advice
from 100 Top Medical Experts

SARI HARRAR

HEARST
books

CONTENTS

INTRODUCTION

The Huge, Simple Secret to Improving Your Weight, Health, Memory, and Energy?

Do What Doctors Do

DOCTORS AREN'T SUPERHUMAN. They aren't bionic. And they weren't born with super-duper immunity or better genes. But the fact is that doctors and other health practitioners enjoy a health edge because of their authoritative knowledge. The American Medical Association recently asked its physicians to get personal. It's time, the AMA told its members, for docs to share their private health secrets with the rest of us. Yet relatively few doctors have gone public with their private health strategies and never all in one place. Until *now*.

This is the book that shows you how more than 100 of America's leading health practitioners stay healthy, happy, energized, and remarkably disease-free. You'll be startled by how simple, doable, and effective their strategies are.

How does clinical psychologist Susan Albers, PhD, of the Cleveland Clinic reduce stress in five minutes? With a "Ho-Ho-Ho" meditation—laughter therapy based on research that shows that giggling and guffawing, even if you *make* yourself laugh, releases feel-good brain chemicals that tame tension. We'll tell you how to do it.

How does Mehmet Oz, MD—host of the award-winning *Dr. Oz Show*, vice chair and professor of surgery at Columbia University, director of the Cardiovascular Institute and Complementary Medicine Program at New York Presbyterian Hospital, founding editor of a new magazine, and the definition of busy doc—set the stage for a healthy day? With "no-brainer" choices that are easy and automatic. No need to use up willpower or waste time deciding! He sets aside seven minutes (!) for a serious but super-efficient exercise routine and *always* has the same breakfast (yogurt and fruit). "You can save energy for the tougher challenges if you make parts of your routine constant," he explains.

How does May Hsieh Blanchard, MD, chief of the division of general obstetrics and gynecology at the University of Maryland School of Medicine in Baltimore, remember to take her vitamins? By keeping a little pillbox beside her toothbrush, she says.

THINK—AND ACT—LIKE A TOP DOC

In extensive interviews, we've uncovered the nine smart, easy steps doctors take for optimal health—things you can use today, *without* going through the nine intense years of medical training it took for them to figure these out!

1 **THEY'VE GOT THE SCIENCE-BASED INSIDE SCOOP ON WHAT WORKS BEST**—and what's a bust. Want to know the ideal coffee "dosing" for staying alert after a late night? How not to catch a cold on an airplane? Which drugstore skincare bargains are worth buying? The real deal on weight-loss surgery? Top docs have science-based answers to these questions. They've even pinpointed the best way to blow your nose. (Really. Getting it wrong only makes things worse, as you'll discover on page 104.)

2 **THEY KNOW HOW TO BE SUPER PRACTICAL,** even if it means wearing sneakers to work or toting around mini bags of baby carrots. Doctors usually have zero extra time, so they go for the stuff that's fast, easy, and really works. And, nope, they're not afraid to look uncool if that's what it takes. They may walk around airports to burn calories instead of hunching over an overpriced beer in a terminal bistro. They often eat the same quick, healthy breakfast *every* day because it means there's one less thing to think about. Many do deep breathing to wind down when they realize they've tensed up.

3 **THEY REGULARLY MIX CONVENTIONAL AND COMPLEMENTARY MEDICINE.** Surprisingly, docs are among the biggest personal users of alternative therapies. They know what delivers (acupressure, meditation, well-chosen herbs) and what doesn't (colonics and cleanses get a big "no thanks").

4 **THEY KNOW WHEN TO ACT FAST.** Ever wonder what top docs keep in *their* first aid kits? How they treat everyday emergencies like a bad kitchen cut or small toaster burn? Their strategies range from high-tech (products that instantly stop bleeding) to down-home (onions for minor burns?!). Either way, they can spring into action if trouble flares. Now, you can be just as prepared with the tips in chapters 8 and 9.

5 **THEY'RE SMART HEALTHCARE CONSUMERS THEMSELVES.** Top docs know that a family health history is more powerful than genetic testing for finding inherited risks. They know—and share—the best way to handle an ER trip, how to get a first-rate second opinion in the middle of nowhere, and the surest way to sidestep the number one prescription error at pharmacies. Soak up their savvy in chapter 11.

6 **THEY *GET* THE TESTS MANY OF US PUT OFF . . . INDEFINITELY.** Blood pressure and cholesterol? Sure. But regular colonoscopies, mammograms, and prostate screenings? Just as sure. Docs know these screenings provide crucial info and can reduce the risk of life-threatening diseases. Find out in chapter 10 why most don't skip even sometimes controversial scheduled tests.

7 **THEY KNOW THAT LITTLE THINGS CAN MAKE A *BIG* DIFFERENCE.** Case in point: healthy food. In chapter 2, you'll discover why a little good fat unlocks the disease-fighting potential of green veggies, why leaving a cinnamon shaker on the kitchen counter could help the entire family's health, and why, if you juice, it's worth baking the leftover fiber into brownies for your kids!

8 **YES, THEY *DO* TAKE SUPPLEMENTS.** In fact, studies show that docs are significantly more likely to take multivitamins and other supplements than the average American—despite having firsthand access to the seemingly endless stream of confusing studies saying this vitamin is still good, that mineral's now bad, and your old reliable's a dud. Which supplements do top docs swear by and why? Check chapter 3.

9 **THEY INDULGE *BECAUSE* IT'S HEALTHY.** Ahhh . . . the good life. It's great for your body as well as your soul. That's one reason why even the busiest docs make time to have fun with friends, indulge in special treats, and kick back with the people they love. They know that many health problems—from heart disease to heartburn—stay away or improve with a little daily R&R and feel-good stress reduction. You'll find dramatic examples in this book—and even specific, fun, healthy ways to let off steam.

Turn the page and get started on the path to better health!

CHAPTER

1

WEIGHT-LOSS SECRETS

ARE ELASTIC-WAIST PANTS AND BIG SHIRTS YOUR STRATEGY
for camouflaging extra pounds? They won't be if you follow the advice
of top docs! Nearly one in three Americans—35% of the adult population—
tips the scales into the obese range—and docs see the human toll obesity
takes every day: soaring odds of heart disease, diabetes, arthritis, and/or cancer.

In this chapter, you'll discover genious ways top docs recommend
avoiding weight gain. It's not magic—everyone faces plenty of waist-widening
challenges these days, like long, stressful workdays that make it tough
to stick with exercise, say no to a sugary afternoon pick-me-up, and grab
fast meals at work, not to mention survive meeting buffets (one headline-
grabbing study found menus offering almost nothing but "rich, sweet,
caloric foods" and desserts at every meal!).

So how do docs recommend doing it? To maintain a healthy weight,
physicians exercise at least twice a week, says a Gallup poll. And docs eat
more of the foods that keep all of us slim—high-fiber/high-satisfaction
fruits, vegetables, and whole grains. They're also less likely than the
average American to sit down to high-calorie fare like fatty meats and
refined carbohydrates.

As obesity rates rise across the nation, take some advice from these
busy physicians. They're the ones *not* shopping for XXXL T-shirts.

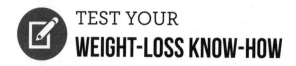

TEST YOUR
WEIGHT-LOSS KNOW-HOW

Almost everyone knows that battling extra pounds isn't easy. So how can you steer clear of the nation's burgeoning obesity epidemic? You're about to find out. Take this test, then read on to discover the research-proven strategies and motivation docs personally rely on to stay slim and trim. Your waistline and your health will thank you!

1 You overindulged at a party last night and woke up feeling miserable and guilty. So for breakfast you:

a. Have a cup of black coffee . . . and swear to ride out the hunger pangs until lunch.

b. Stop at a drive-through for a doughnut and big, creamy coffee drink. What the heck, you've already blown it.

c. Eat a bowl of Cheerios and bananas with your coffee and promise to reform.

2 Juice cleanses are all the rage with celebrities and other trendsetters. Here's what to expect if you try one:

a. A small miracle. You'll lose some weight and improve your health.

b. Anything but a miracle. You'll feel tired, irritable, and maybe even catch a cold.

c. Not much. You may temporarily flatten your belly but the main thing that will slim down is your wallet.

3 Are nuts a brilliant addition to a weight-loss plan . . . or a diet disaster?

a. Brilliant. These fat- and protein-packed nuggets help control overeating.

b. A disaster. Nuts just aren't worth the calories.

c. Nuts are a once-in-a-while splurge when you're taking a vacation from your diet.

4 Which one of these drinks can help you lose more weight?

a. Hot tea

b. One of those nutrient-packed "green drinks"

c. Cold water

5 **True or false:** Top docs never eat large portions.

6 This "naughty" activity can help you lose weight—and keep it off:

a. Running in the nude

b. Gambling

c. Eating only sweets.

FIND THE ANSWERS ON PAGE 28!

SQUELCH OVEREATING WITH NUTS

Thirty minutes before a meal where I think I might overeat, I have six walnut halves. I also munch on a small fistful before I leave work in the evening so I don't overdo dinner.

—**MICHAEL F. ROIZEN**, MD, CHIEF WELLNESS OFFICER AT THE CLEVELAND CLINIC AND CO-AUTHOR OF *YOU: THE OWNER'S MANUAL*

 Walnuts contain two kinds of healthy fats, and a little good fat is a big secret to appetite control. Eating about 70 calories' worth 25 to 30 minutes before a meal ups your body's production of two appetite-controlling hormones (CCK and GLP-1). They tell your brain, "Hey, getting full down here!" Meanwhile, levels of an appetite-stimulating hormone called ghrelin start to back down.

The timing is important, because it takes about 25 minutes for CCK to be released and ghrelin to drop. Once that happens, your body receives the signal that it's eating for pleasure, not for hunger, which helps you naturally eat less. Normally, you finish your meal well before your body's natural fullness signals kick in, and you may eat more than you need to. This strategy gets around that. What's more, having a little fat also slows your stomach from emptying, so you stay full longer.

Not a walnut fan? You can get the same hunger-muting effects by eating 12 almonds, 20 peanuts, or a shot glass of pine nuts. In one study, people who munched on any of these before a meal were less hungry and ate 36% fewer calories when they sat down at the table. While nuts are high in calories, these small portions are just enough to push the "start" button on your body's satisfaction system, so they're calories well spent.

Besides, the healthy plant-based fats they contain are good for your entire cardiovascular system and may cut your risk for blood sugar problems, too. That's not all. Nuts also deliver protein, fiber, and minerals like blood-pressure-soothing magnesium and potassium. Almonds, anyone?

TRULY ENJOY DESSERT

My mother's family is Italian, and most family holidays are all about the food. It's hard to choose! I tend to skip the fill-you-up foods like rolls and appetizers and go for the traditional favorites. Even then, I often take home my favorite sweet instead of eating it at the party.

For example, I look forward each year to an Easter dessert called *Pupa con L'Uova*, which is a beautiful Italian treat that looks like an Easter basket. But I don't eat one at the event. There's so much hustle and bustle that I can't really take my time and savor each bite. So I take one (just one!) home and put it in the refrigerator.

Then I wait for a moment when I'm totally alone and the house is peaceful. I put the *Pupa* in the microwave briefly to warm it up and soften the icing, then I break it into pieces and eat it with a cup of coffee. I can truly eat mindfully and enjoy every single bite.

—SUSAN ALBERS, PSYD, CLINICAL PSYCHOLOGIST AT THE CLEVELAND CLINIC WOOSTER FAMILY HEALTH CENTER AND *NEW YORK TIMES* BEST-SELLING AUTHOR OF *EAT Q: UNLOCK THE WEIGHT-LOSS POWER OF EMOTIONAL INTELLIGENCE*

WHY IT WORKS → It sounds counterintuitive, but choosing and thoroughly enjoying one treat works better than struggling to avoid all of them when you're on vacation, at a special dinner, staring down a tempting buffet, or trying to be good at a holiday feast. Pick a favorite guilty pleasure and take it home instead of eating it there. Then, adds Albers, when you're ready to enjoy it, be sure to sit down and eat in a slow, relaxed way. And use *all* of your senses to focus on the taste, flavor, sight, and sound (crunch, sizzle) of your treat.

EAT BREAKFASTS THAT BLOCK WEIGHT GAIN

A healthy, filling, nutritious—and delicious—breakfast is the ultimate meal for *preventing* weight gain because it keeps you full and energized for hours. One of my favorites on a busy spring or summer morning is a bowlful of muesli. Not the boxed kind from the cereal aisle, but homemade muesli, which takes only minutes to make.

Muesli was invented by the Swiss. It's just rolled oats softened in milk and sprinkled with fruit and nuts, but it turns into a fast, yummy breakfast that's loaded with fiber, protein, nutrients, and healthy fats. Soak the oats in milk for five to 10 minutes in the morning while you get dressed. Or try my easy, make-ahead recipe: In the evening, combine two cups of dry rolled oats, four cups of milk (I like unsweetened vanilla almond milk), one teaspoon cinnamon, and one-half teaspoon pure vanilla extract in a large mixing bowl. Cover and refrigerate overnight.

In the morning, scoop out a serving (about three-quarters cup) and sprinkle it with nuts, seeds, fruit, and even shredded veggies—try some of my favorite combos below.

—DAWN JACKSON BLATNER, RDN, CSSD, AUTHOR OF *THE SUPERFOOD SWAP*

 TRY THESE FRUIT AND NUT COMBOS

✔ Sliced plums, candied ginger, and cashews

✔ Sliced banana, unsweetened cocoa, and walnuts

✔ Shredded carrots, raisins, and pecans

✔ Blackberries, a drizzle of honey, and almonds

✔ Grated zucchini, a little pure maple syrup, and sunflower seeds

 WHY IT WORKS → Even though the nuts and seeds add quite a few calories—add about two tablespoons to your bowl—and don't even think about skipping them. Every calorie pays you back with protein, fiber, and good fats that help control your appetite, improve blood sugar, and lower your risk of both heart disease and (yes!) belly weight.

EAT OUT WITHOUT FILLING OUT

When I eat out, I start my meal with a low-fat veggie soup, such as minestrone, or a salad with dressing on the side. I skip soda and fruit drinks and opt for seltzer with a lemon or lime wedge. If I have an alcoholic beverage, it's just one, and usually white wine spritzer or maybe a Bloody Mary—tomato juice has virtually no calories.

For the main dish, I'll split an entrée with someone and order an extra side or two of veggies. If no one wants to share, I immediately put half on another plate and ask the waitstaff to wrap it up right then. Don't leave it to your stomach to decide. Our eyes are bigger than our stomachs!

—LISA R. YOUNG, PHD, RD, ADJUNCT PROFESSOR IN THE DEPARTMENT OF NUTRITION, FOOD STUDIES, AND PUBLIC HEALTH AT NEW YORK UNIVERSITY AND AUTHOR OF *THE PORTION TELLER PLAN*

 Most restaurants (not just fast-food spots) serve super-sized portions, so we all tend to eat more sugar, saturated fat, and blood-pressure-raising sodium—and fewer vegetables— when we eat out, according to a recent Department of Agriculture survey. And we eat out a lot: Americans get 32% of their daily calories from meals eaten away from home. Extra calories compared to a day of home meals? About 134.

Large portions are a major reason that so many of us gain weight and have trouble losing it. So use these strategies to make portions smaller, and order like a top doc, too: Get grilled chicken or fish, and try to swap white rice or potatoes for a second side of veggies.

PUT YOUR MONEY WHERE YOUR MOUTH IS

I lost 40 pounds by making a diet bet with a friend. We set a target date based on a reasonable weight loss of 1.5 pounds per week. But the stakes were steep: half of our annual income. It worked! We both lost the weight.

Losing weight is, of course, only half the battle. You have to keep it off, too. To do that, I made a maintenance bet of $1,000. If I gained even a pound at a weekly weigh-in, that's what I owed my friend. I didn't gain a thing.

—DEAN S. KARLAN, PHD, PROFESSOR OF ECONOMICS AT YALE UNIVERSITY AND CO-FOUNDER OF THE HEALTH-BET WEBSITE WWW.STICKK.COM

WHY IT WORKS → "When there's something big at stake and you're accountable, you stay focused. There's no wiggle room. You push yourself to stay on track. If eating chocolate cake tonight means you'll lose $10 or $50 or $500 at your next weigh-in, dessert suddenly becomes a lot less attractive," says Karlan.

Research supports this. Putting money on the line has proved to dramatically boost weight-loss success in several studies. At the University of Pennsylvania, dieters who stood to win up to $378 were five times more likely to reach their goals than those with no financial incentives. Fully 50% of the betting group lost 16 pounds in 16 weeks, compared to just 10% of the no-bet group. Want to try it? Bet against a friend or use one of the many online "commitment contract" websites where you can place bets to lose pounds, or stop smoking, or reach other get-healthy goals.

"Dressing clings better to dry greens. Give them a whirl in a salad spinner after washing and you'll find you use less dressing."

— **SHARON FRANKE**, DIRECTOR, GOOD HOUSEKEEPING KITCHEN APPLIANCES AND TECHNOLOGY LAB

TAKE THE GUILT OUT OF INDULGENCES

I'm a cardiovascular physiologist in a cardiac rehab lab *and* have undergone an angioplasty myself, so I make very healthy food choices: grilled fish, lots of fruits and vegetables. But I also have a once-in-a-while small piece of cheesecake, because an occasional treat probably isn't harmful. It's the everyday choices that make the difference.

—BARRY FRANKLIN, PHD, DIRECTOR OF PREVENTATIVE CARDIOLOGY AND CARDIAC REHABILITATION AT WILLIAM BEAUMONT HOSPITAL, ROYAL OAK, MICHIGAN

WHY IT WORKS	→

In a fascinating study that takes the guilt out of once-in-a-while indulgences, researchers from the National Institutes of Health found that daily fluctuations of up to 600 calories only led to small body weight changes—about three pounds over several months. Enjoying a slice of birthday cake, or cheese and crackers with a glass of wine on Friday night, won't pack on the pounds if your average daily calorie intake stays close to whatever level maintains your weight. So don't sweat the occasional treat. The human body can compensate for day-to-day calorie variations.

Other research shows that diet detours even help you stay on track—perhaps by temporarily raising levels of the "I'm full" hormone called leptin. Treats can also cheat-proof your eating plan. In a University of Pittsburgh study that tracked 142 overweight dieters for 11 months, those who took diet breaks lost the same amount of weight as those who dieted nonstop. Researchers suspect the constant dieters cheated more. They needed a break to succeed!

CLOSE YOUR KITCHEN AT 7 P.M.

If you're always trying to maintain a desirable weight—who isn't?—eat a light, early dinner, ideally around 5:30 p.m. but no later than 6:30 or 7:00.

An early-bird dinner hour isn't that unusual for seniors or families with young children, and it has helped me hold the line on my weight. After 7:00 at night, I don't eat at all, although I will drink water or herbal tea.

—LESLIE MENDOZA TEMPLE, MD, MEDICAL DIRECTOR OF THE INTEGRATIVE MEDICINE PROGRAM AT NORTHSHORE UNIVERSITY HEALTHSYSTEM, NEW YORK

 Research backs up the weight benefits of closing your kitchen early in the evening. In a 2013 study at Brigham Young University, volunteers skipped calories between 7 p.m. and 6 a.m. for two weeks, then returned to their usual eating habits.

The result? Not eating at night cut their calorie intake by an average of 238 calories per day. They took in significantly less fat, too, and lost just a bit less than one pound each, without dieting. But when they returned to eating after 7 p.m., they gained an average of 1.3 pounds. As always, the trick is sticking with it.

"When it comes to snacks, keep it real. The tendency to fall back on processed foods is only difficult when you're unprepared. Pack snacks made from real food that isn't 'diet' food: It's food that satisfies both a craving for something indulgent, and staving off the temptation to say 'screw it' and go to McDonald's."

—JACLYN LONDON, MS, RD, GOOD HOUSEKEEPING NUTRITION DIRECTOR

MOVE! FOUR STAY-FIT SECRETS

Want to know my biggest pet diet peeve? People saying I'm slim because I inherited good genes. As anyone over 30 knows, it takes constant work to stay fit and lean in our culture!

What do nutrition pros do to stay fit? We find ways to *stay* active.

 A FEW OF MY TIPS:

▶ **TURN OFF THE TUBE.** Hours of watching TV are directly proportional to weight gain. Go for an after-dinner walk, actually ride your exercise bike (!), do laundry, paint the living room, *move.*

▶ **MAKE EXERCISE FUN.** Listen to books on tape, walk the dog, blast your favorite album and dance, explore new neighborhoods on your bike, change your workouts every season.

▶ **GIVE YOURSELF MINI CHALLENGES.** If you're comfortable walking at a moderate speed, start picking up the pace every few minutes or add some short hills to your route.

▶ **HANG OUT WITH EXERCISERS.** They're incredibly good influences.

—ELIZABETH SOMER, MA, RD, AUTHOR OF MANY BOOKS, INCLUDING *EAT YOUR WAY TO SEXY: REIGNITE YOUR PASSION, LOOK TEN YEARS YOUNGER AND FEEL HAPPIER THAN EVER*

 The most important predictor of whether or not you succeed at permanent weight loss is physical activity. Successful losers are very active, burning about 2,800 calories a week. That's the equivalent of walking four miles a day.

EAT SLOWER, LOSE FASTER

"Slow down—you're eating too fast!" Mothers and diet gurus have been dishing out this admonition for decades. With reason. I try to eat all my meals slowly because it can take up to 15 minutes for the brain to recognize that your stomach is full. Taking your time helps you avoid overeating. Me, too.

—SANJAY GUPTA, MD, CHIEF MEDICAL CORRESPONDENT FOR CNN AND ASSOCIATE CHIEF OF NEUROSURGERY AT ATLANTA'S GRADY MEMORIAL HOSPITAL

 Just a few years ago, researchers tested the hypothesis to see if slow eating actually reins in your appetite. In a University of Rhode Island study, researchers invited 30 women to lunch—twice. Both times they were served huge portions of pasta with tomato sauce and grated Parmesan cheese. On the first visit, the women were asked to eat as quickly as possible. On the second, they were asked to eat slowly, putting down their utensils between bites and chewing each mouthful 15 to 20 times.

When the women ate quickly, they downed 646 calories in nine minutes flat. When they ate slowly, they ate 579 calories in 29 minutes—79 fewer calories. Other research has confirmed that slower eaters tend to eat fewer calories per minute *and* to weigh less.

It's not just that poky diners don't have time to fork up more food. Slowing down gives the brain time to pick up body signals, including the release of the hormone leptin from your fat cells and the compound cholecystokinin from your digestive system. Both of them say, "That's enough. I'm full."

RESET YOUR APPETITE CLOCK

If you're never hungry in the morning, it's likely because you're eating too close to bedtime. If you routinely pass up breakfast, try skipping dinner one night to reset your hunger signals. This will adjust your appetite clock so you'll definitely wake up hungry and break the cycle. Instead of forcing yourself to eat breakfast, now you'll naturally want it.

While some headline-grabbing studies have questioned the importance of breakfast for weight control, there's plenty of evidence that when you eat may be as important as what you eat in terms of maintaining a slim waistline and a healthy weight:

▶ **SKIPPING THE FIRST MEAL OF THE DAY** jumps your obesity risk fourfold, while eating a healthy breakfast lowers the danger of diabetes and insulin problems by 35 to 50%.

▶ **IN A MAJOR 2013 STUDY,** Harvard researchers tracked almost 27,000 men for 16 years. Those who skipped breakfast had a 27% higher risk for a heart attack or fatal heart disease than those who sat down to a morning meal.

▶ **DON'T SKIP BREAKFAST!**

—DAWN JACKSON BLATNER, RDN, CSSD, AUTHOR OF *THE SUPERFOOD SWAP*

 Skipping breakfast makes you crave high-calorie foods later on. In London studies, guys ate a scale-busting 20% more at lunch when they missed their morning meal. So if you're among the 31 million Americans who can't be bothered with breakfast, it's time to change your morning ways.

EAT TO LIVE TO 100

If you make the right food choices, you can enjoy the health and longevity benefits of low-calorie eating without ever feeling deprived.

Do what I do, which is based on everything I've learned from studying some of the world's oldest and healthiest people. I don't watch the amount of fruit, veggies, or beans (legumes) that I eat. In fact, I eat a ton of that stuff! I keep my fridge filled with produce that I enjoy, like chopped pineapple, oranges, and grapes. If I'm hungry, I'll eat half a pound of it. And I know I'll never get fat.

The Okinawa Centenarian Study has uncovered the longevity secrets of 900 people aged 100 or older from Okinawa, Japan, home to one of the world's highest concentrations of *healthy* centenarians. A major finding: These long-lifers have below-average blood levels of free radicals, the rogue oxygen molecules that damage cells and boost your risk of heart disease, cancer, and other major health problems.

—BRADLEY WILLCOX, MD, MS, CO-PRINCIPAL INVESTIGATOR OF THE OKINAWA CENTENARIAN STUDY AND CO-AUTHOR OF *THE OKINAWA DIET PLAN: GET LEANER, LIVE LONGER, AND NEVER FEEL HUNGRY*

 While genes play a role in longevity, researchers suspect that the Okinawa centenarians' traditional Japanese cuisine—low in calories and packed with vegetables, legumes (mostly soybean foods), seafood, and jasmine tea, but with limited red meat and dairy—is the major difference. These foods deliver phytochemicals that help the body disarm free radicals and activate genes, such as FOXO3, responsible for longevity.

"You can make these changes over a few years. I did," says Willcox. "And sure, you can have treats. If you want chocolate, eat a few pieces of dark chocolate that contain about 75 calories apiece. Have a glass of red wine or a beer. But basically try to eat like a traditional Okinawan. I do, and I've lost 20 pounds and am close to my high school weight!"

10-SECOND SOLUTIONS

PECKISH? HAVE A DRINK

"When I'm hungry, I drink some water and wait a bit. Thirst and hunger are easily confused by the body."

—**SANJAY GUPTA,** MD, CHIEF MEDICAL CORRESPONDENT FOR CNN AND ASSOCIATE CHIEF OF NEUROSURGERY AT ATLANTA'S GRADY MEMORIAL HOSPITAL.

BONUS: When 48 overweight adults embarked on low-cal diets for a Virginia Tech study, half drank two cups of water before every meal. Twelve weeks later, the water sippers had lost an average of 15.5 pounds each; the water skippers averaged only an 11-pound loss.

THE SIMPLEST, SHORTEST, HEALTHIEST DIET EVER

"Eat two fruits or vegetables at every meal and one at every snack. You'll easily meet your daily quota of five to nine servings *and* be full, so you'll automatically cut back on fat and calories. Then follow the 25 percent rule: Cut your portions of everything else by one-quarter. Hello, skinny!"

—**ELIZABETH SOMER,** MA, RD, AUTHOR OF MANY BOOKS, INCLUDING *EAT YOUR WAY TO SEXY: REIGNITE YOUR PASSION, LOOK TEN YEARS YOUNGER AND FEEL HAPPIER THAN EVER*

DON'T LET TV MAKE YOU FAT

When one survey asked people how they knew it was time to put down their forks, a surprising number said things like "When my TV show is over." Better idea: Stop when you feel full.

—**BRIAN WANSINK**, PHD, AUTHOR OF *SLIM BY DESIGN: MINDLESS EATING SOLUTIONS FOR EVERYDAY LIFE*

"SALAD CLEANSES" BEAT JUICE CLEANSES

Almost overnight, packaged juice "cleanses" have become a multimillion-dollar industry. Yet these pricey drinks aren't a good choice for dropping pounds or making your belly look more than temporarily flatter. Juice cleanses are expensive and can leave you feeling hungry, tired, and run down. One reason: They don't supply all the nutrients you need. Your immunity can be compromised, too. Instead of jumpstarting a weight-loss resolution, you could get the flu.

Plus, you'll absolutely need supplements to support liver function and get adequate nutrition. Bottom line: A multiday juice cleanse can be dangerous without medical supervision.

—THERI GRIEGO RABY, MD, FOUNDER AND MEDICAL DIRECTOR OF THE RABY INSTITUTE FOR INTEGRATIVE MEDICINE AT NORTHWESTERN UNIVERSITY IN CHICAGO

Instead, when you're feeling bloated and less than svelte, try this far better plan: Do a five-night "salad cleanse." Every evening, have a big salad for supper. Start with a base of hearty greens (kale and spinach are ideal), then top with some lean protein (chickpeas, pork, skinless chicken, beans, tuna, shrimp), plenty of veggies and fruit (roasted red peppers, grilled asparagus, mushrooms, orange sections, raspberries, etc.), and a good fat (a tablespoon of chopped nuts, or a few olives or avocado slices). Top with a tablespoon of vinaigrette made with olive oil, balsamic vinegar, and seasonings of your choice.

WHY IT WORKS → These high-fiber, reduced-calorie "salad cleanse" dinners will kick-start weight loss and encourage great digestion. They're packed with nutrients and other healthy plant substances from juicy fruits and vegetables, plus they're leavened with lean protein and a smidge of healthy fat. Upshot: You'll feel healthy, not ready to keel over. And you'll start liking the scales again.

WEIGHT-LOSS SURGERY IS NO JOKE

When overweight friends ask me about the "quick fix" of bariatric or gastric bypass surgery, I answer, "Don't be fooled by celebrities who make these operations look like the easiest way to ditch pounds. They're not."

Here's the reality: These procedures require your total commitment. You must be willing to work with a psychiatrist and a dietitian. You'll need frequent blood tests post-surgery to make sure you're getting proper vitamins and nutrients. You have to eat all of your foods in small bites, avoid drinking with your meals, and stop eating the *second* you feel full. And you have to do all of that for the rest of your life. Weight-loss surgery is a last resort.

—JAIME PONCE, MD, BARIATRIC SURGEON IN DALTON, GEORGIA, AND PAST PRESIDENT OF THE AMERICAN SOCIETY FOR METABOLIC AND BARIATRIC SURGERY

WHY IT WORKS →

Despite its many drawbacks, if you're committed to making healthy changes for the long haul, weight-loss surgery can help you lose a significant number of pounds—and improve a wide variety of serious health conditions. These include type 2 diabetes, joint pain, sleep apnea, high cholesterol, high blood pressure, and painful circulation problems in the legs. In studies, it has also reduced erectile dysfunction in men and improved fertility in women by correcting some hormone imbalances.

"From vanilla lattes to Frappuccinos, your morning cup of joe could be a sneaky source of added calories. Instead, opt for a skim, soy, or low-fat cappuccino, café au lait, or caffe misto. Even better: Black coffee is a zero-calorie choice. Have to have milk? Always fill your cup with more coffee and skip flavored syrup, sugar, or caramel."

—JACLYN LONDON, MS, RD, GOOD HOUSEKEEPING NUTRITION DIRECTOR

CAN'T LOSE WEIGHT? SUSPECT YOUR THYROID

A friend in my book club who had put on some pounds was working hard to slim down. She was eating well and exercising regularly, but couldn't lose the weight. She asked her doctor if her thyroid might be to blame, but he dismissed the idea. I had no problem saying that her doctor was probably wrong.

In fact, for women over 35 who struggle with excess weight, I live by the rule of "slow thyroid until proven otherwise." My friend got more extensive tests, and lo and behold, she had a sluggish thyroid and more. She was treated not just with a thyroid medication but with multivitamins and vitamin D. Two months later, she was back to her normal, healthy weight.

—**SARA GOTTFRIED**, MD, BOARD-CERTIFIED GYNECOLOGIST, INTEGRATIVE PHYSICIAN, AND AUTHOR OF *THE HORMONE CURE*

 Thyroid issues are one of the most common reasons for a slumping metabolism and slow weight loss. Fatigue, puffiness, feeling cold all the time, depression, and dry hair and skin can all also be signs of an underactive thyroid. About one in 50 adults has full-blown hypothyroidism—marked by high levels of thyroid-stimulating hormone (TSH) and low levels of thyroxine hormone.

But this statistic is even more relevant: As many as one in 20 people—especially women and older adults—has less-obvious subclinical hypothyroidism, which often has no obvious symptoms and requires a blood test to diagnose (it's marked by high TSH but normal thyroxine levels). Weight gain isn't the only concern. It can make you feel sluggish and up your risk for brittle bones and out-of-rhythm heartbeats called atrial fibrillation.

ANSWERS TO
WEIGHT-LOSS KNOW-HOW

1 **C.** Did you know that skipping breakfast increases your odds for obesity fourfold? That's one reason top docs and nutrition experts swear by a filling, nutritious morning meal as their favorite way to ward off overeating later in the day. *See pages 21 and 22.*

2 **B & C.** Top nutrition experts recommend jump-starting a diet with plenty of fruits and vegetables, along with leafy greens, lean protein and some good fats. You get world-class nutrition and reduce belly-bloating problems, too. *See page 25.*

3 **A.** Eating a handful of nuts 25 to 30 minutes before a meal resets key appetite-controlling hormones, dialing down cravings so you eat a little less. *See page 13.*

4 **C.** Sipping two glasses of cool H_2O before a meal fills you up and could help you lose 40% more weight. *See page 24.*

5 **FALSE.** Studying some of the world's healthiest, longest-living people has shown that eating certain foods to your heart's content won't make you fat. *Find out which ones on page 23.*

6 **B.** Want to permanently lose a significant number of pounds? Place a hefty bet on doing it. Gambling on weight loss can make you a winner. How? *See page 17.*

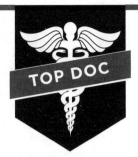

TOP DOC

REMEMBER THESE FIVE WEIGHT-LOSS SECRETS

In this chapter, top docs revealed the weight-control strategies that work, which range from commonsense to quirky. Their experiences illuminate a big truth about weight control: Don't skip the fundamentals—calorie control, exercise, healthy foods. Adapt these strategies to fit your individual needs:

1 **DON'T SKIP MEALS.** You'll just open the door to hunger, cravings, and low energy. A well-chosen meal fuels work and exercise and is an insurance policy against overeating later on.

2 **REBALANCE YOUR PLATE.** Pile on the produce, leave room for whole grains, add a little lean protein and a smidge of good fats. This approach keeps calories under control while supplying plenty of high-satisfaction, high-nutrition foods.

3 **SIP SMART.** Top docs skip high-calorie drinks, including soda, sweet tea, rich coffee drinks, and excess alcohol. They drink plenty of water, known to turbocharge weight-loss diets. H_2O, anyone?

4 **COMBINE DIET AND EXERCISE.** Unless you're training for a marathon or triathlon, don't rely on exercise to eliminate loads of calories. That's what smart eating excels at. What exercise *is* brilliant at: helping you stay on track by slashing stress, boosting feel-good brain chemicals, and building lean, buff muscle. Yes, it burns some calories, but it's mainly these other benefits that make exercise the single strongest predictor of weight-loss success.

5 **FIND YOUR OWN UNIQUE SWEET SPOT.** What one thing would help you diet smarter? Do you need a way to curb overeating at meals? Have trouble sticking with a plan for the long haul? Need a way to fit in the occasional treat, big portion, or "diet vacation" without feeling like you've blown it? Name your need, then apply the top-doc strategy in this chapter that addresses it. You'll be slimmer in no time!

CHAPTER

2

FOODS THAT FIGHT DISEASE

AS A GROUP, doctors think fruits and vegetables are "da bomb." They recommend eating an average of five servings of fruit and vegetables every day, outstripping the average American, who munches just three servings. Doctors recommend a diet that is healthier in other ways, too:

EAT WITH A PURPOSE. Three-quarters of physicians say they recommend following a science-based eating strategy that is *proven* to slash the risk of heart attacks, strokes, and more. Top choices: the American Heart Association's healthy eating plan and the Mediterranean diet (see page 43). Both emphasize fruits and vegetables, lean protein, good fats, and whole grains.

EAT FISH. About 43% of male doctors have fish two to four times a week, and 11% eat fish *five* times a week, reports a Harvard Medical School study that's been tracking 25,000 docs since 1982. Having fish instead of meat lowers your intake of heart-risky saturated fat and often delivers a dose of heart- and brain-friendly omega-3 fatty acids, too.

GO MEATLESS. Vegetarians tend to be slimmer, live longer, and have lower rates of heart disease, diabetes, cancer, and more. Only 2 to 3% of the US population currently eats a vegetarian diet.

EAT MORE WHOLE GRAINS. Physicians consume about one and a half servings of fiber-packed whole grains daily, versus one for the rest of us.

What can help you eat smart *and* stick with it successfully long-term so that you can sidestep fatal heart disease, cancer, and other killers? It comes down to doing lots of little things right, little things you can easily do. They make a *big* difference.

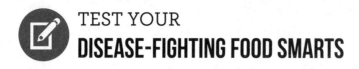

TEST YOUR
DISEASE-FIGHTING FOOD SMARTS

Top docs face the same food choices the rest of us do. But they use their medical experience—and common sense—to maximize the benefits and minimize the downsides when eating at restaurants, shopping at grocery stores, or choosing snacks. Are you food-smart about choosing disease-fighting foods? Take this quiz and find out.

1 Leafy green vegetables contain compounds that help battle cancer, diabetes, and heart disease—but absorption is hampered if you add this to your salad:

a. Cheese

b. Fat-free salad dressing

c. Meat

2 Cutting back on added sugars also helps you prevent diabetes, heart disease, obesity, and more. But to sweeten your tea or a bowl of strawberries, which of these is the healthiest choice?

a. Agave syrup or raw sugar

b. White table sugar or brown sugar

c. Honey

3 **True or false:** If a plastic container is BPA-free, it's safe to microwave food in it.

4 Men should have no more than two alcoholic drinks per day, but women should stick with one. Why the difference?

a. Women are smaller than men.

b. Women's bodies make less of the enzyme that breaks down alcohol.

c. Alcohol raises breast cancer risk.

5 A growing stack of research suggests that diet soda encourages weight gain and ups the risk of diabetes and heart disease. Why?

a. Its artificial ingredients take a slow but steady health toll.

b. It encourages "magical thinking" about calories.

c. The carbonation is bad for you.

6 **True or false:** Dairy products are now thought to be bad for your bones.

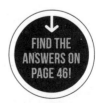

FIND THE ANSWERS ON PAGE 46!

EAT GREEN VEGGIES LIKE THERE'S NO TOMORROW

The best foods you can eat to keep your immune system strong are green vegetables. They're loaded with disease-fighting antioxidants, which also keep aging free radicals in your body under control. My fridge is always stocked with lettuces, broccoli, and kale. They're my secret weapons during flu season, and I rely on them all year long to fend off cancer, heart disease, type 2 diabetes, and other chronic conditions. Enough said.

—**JOEL FUHRMAN**, MD, RESEARCH DIRECTOR OF THE NUTRITIONAL RESEARCH FOUNDATION IN FLEMINGTON, NEW JERSEY, AND AUTHOR OF *THE END OF HEART DISEASE*, AMONG OTHER BOOKS

JUST ONE TIP: Skip fat-free salad dressings. To get the most nutrients out of green salads, your body needs the heart-healthy good fats from whole nuts and seeds, such as walnuts, almonds, or sesame seeds. They can be blended in to make delicious dressings and help your system absorb the carotenoids and other protective phytochemicals in raw greens.

 WHY IT WORKS → **WHAT MAKES GREEN VEGGIES SO POWERFUL?**

▶ They have more micronutrients per calorie than all other foods.

▶ They help weight control because they're low-cal and rich in filling fiber.

▶ Their antioxidants and protective plant compounds called phytochemicals activate something called Nrf2—a factor that aids your body's natural detoxification system.

▶ They may help shield your arteries from harmful inflammation and stiffness.

▶ They contain two carotenoids called lutein and zeaxanthin—which your body can't make itself—that protect against cataracts and age-related macular degeneration. Lutein may also fight heart disease.

STR-R-R-ETCH THAT COCKTAIL

Enjoying alcohol in moderation can be a challenge on a long evening out, especially for women because "moderation" means one drink. For men it means two. Why the difference? One is that women have lower levels of the alcohol-metabolizing enzyme alcohol dehydrogenase. So when a man and a woman who are exactly the same size have exactly the same drink, the woman's blood alcohol levels can be up to 30% higher. Over time, that makes the alcohol far more likely to damage her brain, pancreas, liver, heart, and breasts.

One strategy I use on nights out is to befriend the bartender (and tip!) and request a favor: Ask him or her to stretch your cocktail order into three separate servings over the course of the night. Another approach: Start the evening with iced tea or soda, have one drink later on, then switch back to soft drinks before you leave. Whatever works!

—SUZANNE THOMAS, PHD, ASSOCIATE PROFESSOR OF PSYCHIATRY AT THE MEDICAL UNIVERSITY OF SOUTH CAROLINA AND RESEARCHER AT THE SCHOOL'S CHARLESTON ALCOHOL RESEARCH CENTER

WHY IT WORKS → Let's say you drink vodka tonics and ask the bartender to stretch them. Each glass will contain mostly tonic water and ice, with one-third of a normal serving of vodka. That means you can have three drinks and still consume only one serving of alcohol (1.5 ounces of 80-proof liquor). A similar approach can be used with white wine: Have the bartender mix it with lots of seltzer to make three light wine spritzers.

Plan C, says Thomas: "Order your drink neat and request an extra-large glass of water, tonic, or soda. Add your drink to the large glass and sip throughout the night."

TRADE UP TO HEALTHIER FOOD

Learning to love the foods that love you back gives you the pleasure of good eating *and* good health. All that stands in the way is your taste buds' familiarity with the status quo. But you can put your taste buds in "rehab" and see changes quickly. I've done it myself.

The trick is to gradually trade up. Make healthier choices in every category. Start by trading up to foods lower in added salt, sugar, and fat—for instance, choose whole grains instead of refined grains. If you're already eating whole-grain breads, pasta, and cereal, trade up to even less-refined grains—have steel-cut oats for breakfast, a side of barley or brown rice with dinner. Instead of juice, choose whole fruit. Instead of chips, have crunchy sliced veggies. Instead of ice cream, have a bowl of beautiful berries.

—**DAVID L. KATZ**, MD, MPH, FACPM, FACP, FOUNDING DIRECTOR OF YALE UNIVERSITY'S PREVENTION RESEARCH CENTER, PRESIDENT OF THE AMERICAN COLLEGE OF LIFESTYLE MEDICINE, AND AUTHOR OF *DISEASE-PROOF: THE REMARKABLE TRUTH ABOUT WHAT MAKES US WELL*

 WHY IT WORKS → "The science is clear and convincing: Your taste buds are excellent adapters. They happily learn to love the foods they're with when they're no longer with the foods they used to love," says Katz. Just as eating junkier, saltier, fattier, sweeter, more-processed foods teaches your taste buds to prefer them, eating more fresh, delicious, nutritious food trains them to prefer the good stuff. And with every trade-up, you cut out gobs of sugar, fat, and sodium—while adding fiber, antioxidants, and more. Your body will thank you a hundred times over.

SNACK
WITH A PURPOSE

How do I get calcium? I have a 12-ounce skim latte every day. I also snack on low-fat cheese sticks and treat myself to frozen yogurt at night. All three are full of calcium, which is key for muscle function and bone health.

I am a strong believer in getting nutrition from food when possible. Calcium tablets provide calcium in a form that is not absorbed well. In contrast, calcium-packed dairy products also provide some natural carbohydrates along with vitamin D, potassium, magnesium, and lots of protein. Plus they taste good! I shoot for four to five servings of dairy products a day. My favorite frozen yogurt treat? French vanilla with chocolate chips sprinkled on top. Yum.

—SHARON PHELAN, MD, FACOG, PROFESSOR OF OBSTETRICS AND GYNECOLOGY AT THE UNIVERSITY OF NEW MEXICO SCHOOL OF MEDICINE, ALBUQUERQUE

WHY IT WORKS → Despite some controversies about the benefits of dairy products for bones, plenty of research points to bone and other health payoffs from low- or no-fat milk, yogurt, and cheese. Calcium plus potassium and magnesium are crucial for healthy blood pressure. A University of South Carolina analysis of 17,030 Americans found that people who got more calcium from food had smaller increases in systolic blood pressure as they aged. The Institute of Medicine recommends most adults get at least 1,000 milligrams of calcium a day primarily from food—that's the amount you get in three to four dairy servings.

BE FUSSY ABOUT WHAT GOES IN YOUR MICROWAVE

We're not talking about food. We're talking about containers. Plastic containers. Heat releases some of the chemical building blocks in plastic and can send them into whatever food or drink you're warming up. One chemical, bisphenol A—the now infamous BPA—created a major scare a few years ago when it was found that BPA can "mimic the effects of estrogen in the body, potentially leading to issues like premature puberty and breast or testicular cancer."

—SUZANNE PHAM, MD, PREVENTIVE MEDICINE EXPERT IN CHICAGO, ILLINOIS

WHY IT WORKS → While BPA is mostly gone from plastic containers, it's still in some that have the recycling numbers 3 or 7 on the bottom, says the FDA. But here's the bigger point: Even BPA-free plastics can release substances that could have iffy health effects, so avoid microwaving food in *any* plastic container, says Jennifer Lowry, MD, a medical toxicologist at Children's Mercy Hospitals and Clinics in Kansas City, Missouri. Heat food or drinks in glass or ceramic containers only.

"Be fussy about what goes in your microwave. Glass containers with a tight-fitting lid will do the best job of keeping air out and preserving the life of your food. But do make sure you vent the lid to let some steam escape and avoid steam burns when you remove the cover. If you use plastic wrap as a lid in the microwave, don't let it come in direct contact with food. Instead of plastic wrap, use a paper towel or a paper plate as a lid."

—SHARON FRANKE, DIRECTOR, GOOD HOUSEKEEPING KITCHEN APPLIANCES AND TECHNOLOGY LAB

DOUBLE YOUR DAILY DISEASE DEFENSES

Your grocery cart should always be loaded with colorful fruits and vegetables. Mine is. Why? While we don't know what an "optimal dose" of these foods is, we do know that the more of them you eat, the more you boost your disease defenses. It's hard to overdo. Here are a few ways I trick myself into getting eight to 10 servings of produce a day. Yes, *every* day!

—**ELIZABETH SOMER**, MA, RD, AUTHOR OF MANY BOOKS, INCLUDING *EAT YOUR WAY TO SEXY: REIGNITE YOUR PASSION, LOOK TEN YEARS YOUNGER AND FEEL HAPPIER THAN EVER*

1. **BRING IT:** Always stuff your purse/briefcase/backpack/diaper bag with apples, bananas, mini carrots, and boxes of raisins so you don't wind up staring at a candy counter.

2. **DOUB IT:** This one's super simple. Have a whole grapefruit, not a half. Put twice as many veggies on your dinner plate. Double your salad serving. Done.

3. **HIDE IT:** Stir prunes, berries, or pear chunks into muffins; sprinkle diced dates or dried cranberries on cereal or rice dishes.

4. **CROSS-DRESS IT:** Please your appetite chemicals by combining fruit with sweet treats—dunk strawberries in chocolate syrup, sprinkle crystalline ginger over mandarin oranges, top kiwi slices with berry sorbet.

 WHY IT WORKS → Thousands of studies spanning decades of research consistently show that a diet rich in colorful vegetables and fruit lowers your risk for most age-related diseases—cancer, diabetes, heart disease, hypertension, cataracts, and on and on.

Let bright, eye-catching colors and dark leafy greens be your guide. Think raspberries and sweet potatoes, red cabbage and green kale, pomegranates and plums. The more deeply colored the fruits and vegetables, the more disease-fighting nutrients are likely to be inside them—and to get inside you.

HOME BAKERS, BUMP UP THE FIBER!

I use *white* whole-wheat flour in recipes that call for flour. It tastes like regular white flour, but because it's made with whole grains, I get the added heart-healthy, belly-filling benefits of its extra fiber.

—LISA AIRAN, MD, AESTHETIC DERMATOLOGIST IN NEW YORK CITY AND FORMER NATIONAL INSTITUTES OF HEALTH FELLOW

If you love to bake but the only flour in your cupboard is ordinary white or regular whole wheat, you're about to discover a delicious, super-healthy treat: baked goods made from flours ground from an amazing variety of grains, nuts, seeds, and even beans. They add fiber, nutrition, and super flavor to your favorite baked goods and are now available in some supermarkets and most natural food stores.

Bump up your fiber quotient by trying some of the flours below. This is just a sampling; you'll find more. Be adventurous! Most have directions for substituting them for regular flours.

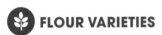 **FLOUR VARIETIES**

▶ **GRAIN FLOURS:** Try barley, oatmeal, and brown rice flours, or ancient grains like protein-rich amaranth, sorghum, and spelt.

▶ **BEAN FLOURS:** Soy's a natural, but you'll find flour from chickpeas, black beans, and other legumes, too. They're a good source of protein and slow-digesting carbohydrates.

▶ **NUT AND SEED FLOURS:** Baking with almond or hazelnut flour adds moisture as well as wonderful flavor; flaxseed flour infuses healthy omega-3 fatty acids.

> **WHY IT WORKS** → The reason doctors and nutritionists make such a big deal about fiber is that most of us get only about half of the 20 to 25 grams of fiber we need daily. This important stuff comes in two varieties. *Insoluble* fiber, the kind in whole wheat, helps you feel full and improves digestion. *Soluble* fiber, found in barley, oats, and beans, helps keep blood sugar and cholesterol levels healthy.

THREE SUGAR MYTHS

MYTH 1: NATURAL SUGARS ARE BETTER FOR YOU.

If only. Agave, honey, cane, brown, raw sugar . . . natural or not, eat too much and you'll gain weight, boost your blood sugar, increase your risk of heart disease, and more. Check label ingredients for sugar under its many names, including molasses, evaporated cane juice, fruit juice concentrates, and anything ending with ose, such as dextrose or maltose. Minimize them all. One type of sugar isn't much healthier than any other.

—**MONICA REINAGEL**, MS, LN, NUTRITIONIST IN BALTIMORE, MARYLAND

MYTH 2: FOCUS ON THE SUGAR IN YOUR SPOON.

It's not the spoonful of sugar in your coffee that's the culprit. It's the sugar hiding in places you don't expect. Sugar is added to 80% of all packaged foods, even things that don't seem sweet, such as pepperoni and savory crackers.

—**NICOLE AVENA,** PHD, SUGAR RESEARCHER AT THE UNIVERSITY OF FLORIDA'S CENTER FOR ADDICTION RESEARCH AND EDUCATION AND AUTHOR OF *WHY DIETS FAIL (BECAUSE YOU'RE ADDICTED TO SUGAR)*

MYTH 3: JUST AVOID HIGH-FRUCTOSE CORN SYRUP AND YOU'LL BE OKAY.

Nope. High-fructose corn syrup may be the most controversial sugar, but at the end of the day, sugar is sugar. It doesn't matter what kind it is. It's quantity that's the problem. When you're comparing food labels, choose the one with the fewest grams of total sugar.

—**MELISSA JOY DOBBINS**, MS, RDN, CDE, SOUND BITES COMMUNICATIONS

EASY RULES FOR THE HEALTHIEST DIET

Remember three simple concepts when you shop for groceries, make a meal, grab a snack, or order in a restaurant: balance, moderation, and variety, advises Richard Mattes, MPH, PhD, RD, distinguished professor of nutrition and director of the Ingestive Behavior Research Center at Indiana's Purdue University. Balance and variety ensure that you get a wide spectrum of nutrients, which research shows contributes to better health. And moderation isn't boring—when you stick with healthy portion sizes, there's room for the occasional guilt-free treat, too.

 It's not just the empty calories. Downing too much refined sugar can trigger an accumulation of fat inside your liver—a major health hazard. It can make your liver sick, threaten your heart, drive up blood pressure, increase your risk of diabetes, and lead to cancer.

—ROBERT H. LUSTIG, MD, MSL, OBESITY EXPERT AT THE UNIVERSITY OF CALIFORNIA SAN FRANCISCO AND AUTHOR OF *FAT CHANCE: BEATING THE ODDS AGAINST SUGAR, PROCESSED FOOD, OBESITY, AND DISEASE*

10-SECOND SOLUTIONS

USE CINNAMON WITH ABANDON

Cinnamon may have benefits beyond jazzing up your breakfast toast or favorite hot cereal, says a recent review in the *Annals of Family Medicine*. Regular users of the loved spice have declines in bad LDL cholesterol and triglycerides—two big heart-disease threats. Cinnamon lovers also get a slight boost in their good HDL cholesterol and it helps keep blood sugar levels steady, which means fewer sugar rushes and hunger pangs throughout the day.

The daily "dose"? While there's no official recommendation for this spice yet, experts recommend sticking with the amount you might get from food in a day—one-half to one teaspoon. Talk to your doctor before taking larger amounts, including supplements.

DRINK YOUR TEA STRAIGHT

The good news: Antioxidant-rich black tea has been shown to significantly improve the functioning of blood vessels. The bad news, especially for Brits and others who like their tea "white": A study in the *European Heart Journal* found that adding milk basically cancels out tea's heart-healthy benefits. The researchers suspect that the milk proteins bind with the tea's antioxidants, neutralizing their effects. What about using soy milk instead? Nope. Its proteins have exactly the same effect.

SEA SALT IS . . . SALT

"Sea salt is no different from table salt in how much sodium it contains," says Melinda Johnson, RD, MS, RDN, clinical assistant professor and didactic program in dietetics director, School of Nutrition and Health Promotion, at Arizona State University. "There's no benefit to buying snacks and other foods that contain sea salt instead of table salt." Other than looking hipper. So whether it's from the sea or the salt mines, limit overall sodium intake to 2,300 mg per day, or 1,500 per day if you're over age 50, African American, or have *high blood pressure, diabetes, or kidney disease.*

SNEAK FIBER INTO KIDS' TREATS

I eat plenty of whole fruits and veggies, and I also juice fresh vegetables and fruits in a cold press. Fresh juice is a great way to get even more vitamins, minerals, and phytonutrients into your diet. As for the leftover fiber, I eat some, cook with some, and bake some into brownies and feed them to my unsuspecting children. Beet fiber is great for this!

—**LESLIE MENDOZA TEMPLE**, MD, MEDICAL DIRECTOR OF THE INTEGRATIVE MEDICINE PROGRAMS AT NORTHSHORE UNIVERSITY HEALTHSYSTEM, NEW YORK

DON'T INHERIT A STROKE

Even if strokes run in your family, the tasty, healthy Mediterranean diet can virtually *eliminate* your increased genetic risk of stroke, reports a 2013 study from Spain. On the Mediterranean menu: moderate amounts of wine, low consumption of meat and meat products, and high intake of vegetables, fruits, nuts, legumes, fish, and olive oil.

—**RAMON ESTRUCH**, MD, PHD, OF MADRID'S INSTITUTO DE SALUD CARLOS III

ALL ABOUT GINGER

"It's time to stock up on this flavorful root. Not only does ginger help soothe joints, but it also helps an upset stomach and may improve our body's insulin sensitivity, which can help reduce inflammation caused by high insulin levels in the blood. Since ginger can be used in sweet and savory dishes, try adding ginger to fruit salads, Asian-inspired sautés, and homemade smoothies. Not a fan of it in your food? Try it in your tea or finely chopped up in a smoothie."

—**JACLYN LONDON**, MS, RD, GOOD HOUSEKEEPING NUTRITION DIRECTOR

HOW TO FLY PAST AIRPORT FOOD TRAPS

I'm borderline obsessive when it comes to packing smart travel snacks—even more so since I had my kids, who are now six and two. Nothing drives me crazier than seeing people load up on fatty, salty, sugary junk food at the airport.

Even more frustrating is the poor selection of healthful snacks on the plane, which often contain several servings per container. You could easily consume more than 500 calories, if you're mindlessly munching while watching a movie or reading a book. Combine that with a can of soda or juice and you've eaten an entire meal's worth of calories while strapped in a seat and burning almost no calories!

When traveling, I always bring a large sliced apple, a 100-calorie pack of almonds (about 17 nuts), a protein bar, and an empty water bottle that I fill at the fountain after going through security. Staying hydrated is really important, and it helps keep your metabolism humming! For longer trips, I sometimes add a turkey sandwich on whole-wheat bread or turkey jerky and a bag of baby carrots.

—MELINA B. JAMPOLIS, MD, INTERNIST AND PHYSICIAN NUTRITION SPECIALIST IN PRIVATE PRACTICE IN LOS ANGELES, CALIFORNIA

> **WHY IT WORKS** → Protein is a great travel snack because it keeps you full and keeps your blood sugar stable. That's why 100-calorie packs of almonds are so good: They have about four grams of protein and almost no saturated fat. Well-chosen protein bars deliver, too; just watch out for candy-bar quantities of sugar. Use Jampolis's 10/10 rule: "Pick bars with at least 10 grams of protein and less than 10 grams of sugar."

MEAT ISN'T EVIL

A juicy burger, a spicy bowl of three-bean chili, or slices of roast chicken for Sunday dinner. However you like it, protein is uniquely satisfying. But it's gotten uniquely confusing, too. The rise of low-carb, high-protein diets might make you think more is better . . . while news about cancer connections to high-fat red meats might not.

You need protein to make muscles, skin, cartilage, bones, blood, and more. And high-protein foods are also key sources of iron, zinc, magnesium, and B vitamins. Meat is an excellent source of protein, with about 21 grams per serving. While worldwide studies have repeatedly linked *fatty* red meat, cold cuts, sausages, and pepperoni with cancer, it's okay to eat a variety of lean meats—emphasis on *lean*—even certain cuts of steak. While chicken is a skinny source of protein, meat has nutritional benefits, too, and keeps your diet interesting and satisfying, says Monica Reinagel, MS, LN, a Baltimore nutritionist. "Pork tenderloin and flank steak are quite lean," she adds.

Also, you may want to reconsider dark-meat chicken. Turns out, the leg and thigh meat have only about 35 more calories per three-ounce serving than chicken breast—and dark meat is a rich source of taurine, an amino acid that may help decrease heart-disease risk in women with high cholesterol, found a study from New York University School of Medicine. Just continue to skip the skin; it has most of the saturated fat.

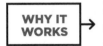 Eating a total of four ounces per day of lean red meat as part of a healthy diet actually *improved* cholesterol levels in one small trial. But to date, no major studies have confirmed this effect and years of research argue against it, so don't go wild. Three ounces (about the size of a deck of cards) is about how much meat should be on your plate. Choose 95% lean ground beef and lean cuts, which typically contain the word "round," as in top round, or "loin," as in tenderloin. And don't make an everyday thing of it. Top docs don't.

ANSWERS TO
DISEASE-FIGHTING FOOD SMARTS

1 **B.** Your digestive system needs some good fat in order to absorb the carotenoids in raw greens, so pass up fat-free dressing and toss your salad with the heart-healthy fats found in an olive or canola oil-based vinaigrette. Adding a few nuts or some avocado to your bowl will also do the trick. *See page 33.*

2 **NONE OF THE ABOVE!** All sugars add calories and, used with abandon, all will send your blood sugar soaring, even those touted as "healthy" or "alternative." Moderation is the key. Don't worry about a teaspoon of sugar. Its 16 calories— enough to sweeten your tea—won't cause trouble for most people. But a can of soda's 14 teaspoons of sugar? That's trouble, and that's why they call it liquid candy. *See page 40.*

3 **FALSE.** Thanks to a flurry of research and headlines, today the health dangers of the plastics additive BPA (bisphenol A) are well known. It's gone from most plastic containers. But that doesn't mean all remaining plastics are microwave-safe. So microwave *only* in glass or ceramic containers. *See page 37.*

4 **B—MAINLY.** Thanks to women's significantly lower levels of the enzyme dehydrogenase, a single drink can make their blood alcohol level 30% higher than that of a man who's the same height and weight. But because alcohol can increase breast cancer risk, some experts urge women at risk of breast cancer to have less than one drink. Also, alcohol's negative effects can be more intense in very small-bodied women. *See page 34.*

5 **B.** Yes, you'll save 150 calories or more when you choose a diet drink over a sugary regular soda. But don't let faulty calorie math tempt you to magically "balance" your calorie savings with a splurge like fries and cookies. *See page 40.*

6 **PROBABLY FALSE.** Despite the bad rap dairy's gotten, there's plenty of evidence that getting about 1,000 milligrams of calcium per day, mostly from food, keeps bones stronger and helps lower fracture risk. You can get calcium from leafy greens, nuts, and tofu, but nothing beats dairy for big doses of this bone-friendly mineral, which supports muscles and healthy blood pressure, too. *See page 36.*

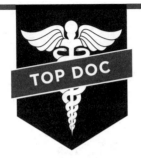

TOP DOC

REMEMBER THIS SMART DISEASE-FIGHTING ADVICE

Eating like a top doc has its advantages— and as you discovered in this chapter, that includes a powerful ability to fend off all kinds of diseases, from flu and bone fractures to Alzheimer's and cancer. To stay as disease-free as many top docs, upgrade your dietary defenses by following these five action steps:

1 **BEING "NATURAL" DOESN'T AUTOMATICALLY MAKE FOOD GOOD.** Natural syrups and raw sugars are as hard on your body as table sugar. Sea salt has no special health benefits. And not all produce has to be 100% organic.

2 **ALWAYS SAVE ROOM IN YOUR PURSE, POCKET, OR BRIEFCASE FOR A HEALTHY SNACK.** Bring along fruit, nuts, mini carrots, even a homemade sandwich when you know you're likely to get hungry and find yourself staring at candy stands, deep-fried mall food, vending-machine fare, or airport grab-n-go shops. Make putting together a healthy snack part of your morning routine.

3 **GIVE YOUR TASTE BUDS A CHANCE TO LOVE SOMETHING NEW.** Worried you'll never truly savor fruit for dessert, extra veggies at dinner, or meatless-Monday bean chili? Have faith. Research shows that taste buds really can change—which really means you can retrain your brain to savor healthy stuff. Just stick with it!

4 **PUT MOSTLY PLANTS ON YOUR PLATE.** The easiest way to eat more fruit, vegetables, and whole grains is by giving them most of the real estate on your plate—think half to produce, one-quarter to grains. Lean protein makes up the rest.

5 **MAKE "HEALTHY INDULGENCE" YOUR NEW MOTTO.** Good eating isn't about steamed broccoli and plain brown rice. Top your salad with a delicious mustard vinaigrette. Spoon up some frozen yogurt to help hit your daily calcium quotient. Look beyond apples and bananas—splurge on berries, juicy melons, and luscious peaches for an irresistible fruit salad. Have some lean beef or pork occasionally and control the portion by grilling skewers of chunks and veggies.

VITAMINS, MINERALS & MORE

NOBODY EATS THE PERFECT DIET DAY IN, DAY OUT. Like the rest of us, docs sometimes skip meals, fuel up at a drive-through, make it through the day (or night) on vending-machine fare, and kick back on Friday night at a casual-dining spot. Like many Americans, almost half (45%) said they eat out at least once a week and 10% acknowledged going for fast food, according to a 2014 national survey that pulled back the curtain on the lifestyles of 30,000 American docs.

That's real life. Doctors know there are nutritional holes in their eating plans, so they fill the gaps with carefully chosen supplements. Their top choices: vitamin D, calcium, omega-3 fatty acids, and multivitamins. Yes, these scientists know all about the controversies over whether multivitamins do much. Yes, many are sticking with their multis.

In fact, when two other recent surveys asked physicians about their use of multivitamins and other dietary supplements, 37% of cardiologists, 50% of orthopedists, and 59% of dermatologists said they were regular users and recommended the same regime to their patients. Over 70% of all docs surveyed took supplements occasionally. So did 74% of dietitians, to bolster bone health, to plug nutritional gaps, and for overall health and wellness.

In this section, you'll get the insider info on what, why, when, and how much top docs recommend you take.

TEST YOUR
SUPPLEMENT SMARTS

Is a multivitamin with iron smarter than an ordinary one? Is calcium helpful or harmful? Can you get all the D you need from the sun? Questions like these likely run through your mind every time you visit the supplement aisle, especially when news stories break about surprising new benefits or scary new risks—and then get contradicted. Top docs cut through the confusion and make confident choices for themselves. Can you? Test your knowledge with this quiz.

1 **True or false:** Multivitamins are not worth taking.

2 **You can get all the vitamin D you need by:**
a. Going outdoors when the sun is shining
b. Eating plenty of D-rich foods
c. Taking a vitamin D supplement

3 **There are three types of omega-3 fatty acids, and all can be found in supplements. Which one is most important for brain and memory health?**
a. ALA
b. DHA
c. EPA

4 **Who should talk with their doctor about taking a vitamin B12 supplement?**
a. Anyone over age 50
b. People taking heartburn drugs
c. Vegetarians

5 **True or false:** Unlike large doses of vitamin A and some others, big doses of vitamin C are safe.

6 **The best time to take a probiotic supplement is:**
a. When you have diarrhea from taking an antibiotic
b. If you want to lose weight
c. Every day—"good bugs" are good for you!

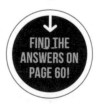

FIND THE ANSWERS ON PAGE 60!

TAKE MULTIVITAMINS

If you have a good, healthy diet—which includes, among other things, eating lots of cruciferous vegetables but not a lot of meat—then you're getting most of the nutrients you need. But the majority of people don't eat this way. That's why I think a good multivitamin is the best place to start.

—JOSEPH MAROON, MD, PROFESSOR OF NEUROSURGERY AT THE UNIVERSITY OF PITTSBURGH AND AUTHOR OF *THE LONGEVITY FACTOR*

 The USDA says most Americans still consume too few fruits, vegetables, whole grains, seafood, and low-fat dairy foods, all of which are crucial to getting enough essential vitamins, minerals, and other nutrients. Other recent studies show that taking a multi has several specific benefits.

1. **CANCER.** Multivitamins can reduce the risk for nonprostate cancers by 8% and the risk for polyps—growths that can morph into colon cancer—by 20%, according to two major American and British studies.

2. **VISION.** If your multi contains 500 mg of vitamin C, 400 IU of vitamin E, 25 mg of zinc, and 2 mg of copper, it helps protect your eyes against low vision and age-related macular degeneration, says research by the National Eye Institute. Lutein (10 mg), zeaxanthin (2 mg), and omega-3 fatty acids (350 mg DHA/650 mg EPA) are also recommended.

3. **FUTURE CHILDREN.** And if you're a woman who might become pregnant, taking both a multi that contains folic acid and an omega-3 fatty acid supplement can dramatically reduce a future baby's risk of birth defects and childhood cancers, explains Michael Roizen, MD, chief wellness officer at the Cleveland Clinic.

Check the label to be sure you're getting 70 to 100% of most vitamins and minerals—but not more. Mega-doses aren't helpful. Your multi should contain the following, but be sure to discuss with your doctor if you have any conditions that prevent your body from processing any of these nutrients:

VITAMINS: A (at least half of it as beta-carotene or mixed carotenoids), B1 (thiamine), B2 (riboflavin), B3 (niacin), B5 (pantothenic acid), B6 (pyridoxine), B7 (biotin), B9 (folic acid), B12, C, D, E, and K.

MINERALS: Copper, chromium, some magnesium, manganese, molybdenum, selenium, zinc, and some calcium. Calcium is too bulky to jam into a multi, so get it from a separate supplement.

FIND A VITAMIN D SWEET SPOT

If you get at least 20 minutes of sun exposure daily on your face, neck, arms, and shoulders (no sunscreen), you may not need a supplement because your skin makes vitamin D when sunlight hits it. You also may not need extra vitamin D if you consume D-fortified milk, yogurt, and breakfast cereals pretty much every day.

But most people do need a supplement. If you live anywhere north of an imaginary line running roughly between San Francisco and Richmond, Virginia—which I do in Connecticut—you just aren't exposed to enough strong sunlight to make the D you need, especially in the fall and winter. Ditto if you're over 70; age slows your skin's D production.

In 2010, the official vitamin D recommendations were tripled. The Institute of Medicine now recommends 600 IU of D daily for kids and adults (800 IU after age 70), but many experts believe that's still not high enough. I also think a little more than that is advantageous. I routinely recommend 1,000 IU a day for most people year-round. It's enough to get the job done but not enough to be dangerous. It's in that sweet spot.

I personally take 1,000 IU daily in the summer and 2,000 IU daily in winter. I go higher for myself in winter because the sun's ultraviolet rays are even weaker and I spend less time outdoors. But if you're thinking about taking more, talk it over with a health professional.

—DAVID L. KATZ, MD, MPH, FACPM, FACP, FOUNDING DIRECTOR OF YALE UNIVERSITY'S PREVENTION RESEARCH CENTER, PRESIDENT OF THE AMERICAN COLLEGE OF LIFESTYLE MEDICINE, AND AUTHOR OF *DISEASE-PROOF: THE REMARKABLE TRUTH ABOUT WHAT MAKES US WELL*

 "Vitamin D is important for immune function, strong bones, cancer prevention, maintaining healthy blood pressure, and possibly reducing your risk of type 1 diabetes," says Katz. Vitamin D also regulates your body's absorption of calcium from food; that's why it's so important for bones, which crave calcium. Recent evidence suggests that sufficient D throughout life may also help prevent colon cancer, cardiovascular disease, and autoimmune disorders.

FIGHT ALZHEIMER'S WITH OMEGA-3S

I routinely take a multi, extra vitamin D, and some calcium. But the thing I'm passionate about taking is my DHA omega-3 supplement. My mother died from complications of Alzheimer's, and I have scoured the research looking for ways to fend off this nasty disease. The DHA form of omega-3 fatty acids is the most promising nutrient I've found.

A wealth of research is accumulating on the brain benefits of DHA. The brain is full of omega-3 fats, and 97% of them are the DHA type. They're critical for normal brain development and function from infancy through your senior years. Some studies indicate that healthy amounts may lower Alzheimer's risk by up to 60%.

The best food sources of DHA are cold-water fatty fish, like salmon, mackerel, tuna, and sardines. Eat them twice a week and you cut the risk of developing memory loss by 28%, according to a study at Tufts. But compared to supplements, they're often expensive and laced with pesticides and mercury.

—**ELIZABETH SOMER**, MA, RD, AUTHOR OF MANY BOOKS, INCLUDING *EAT YOUR WAY TO SEXY: REIGNITE YOUR PASSION, LOOK TEN YEARS YOUNGER, AND FEEL HAPPIER THAN EVER*

WHY IT HELPS → Even for those who love wild salmon and other fish rich in DHA omega-3s, it isn't always easy to get the two to three servings a week needed to provide plenty of DHA, and the toxin levels in fish are a worry. That's why many omega-3 experts take supplements made from DHA-rich algae—it's where fish get their DHA. You can also find foods fortified with algae-based DHA, including some eggs, milk, yogurt, and whole grains.

TAKE CALCIUM THE SAFEST WAY

If you eat a fair amount of green leafy vegetables and dairy foods, you're getting plenty of calcium. So to me, 500 mg a day is enough as a supplement. You want a supplement, not a replacement.

—JOHN PAN, MD, FOUNDER OF THE GEORGE WASHINGTON UNIVERSITY CENTER FOR INTEGRATIVE MEDICINE

Once considered the go-to supplement for strong bones, worries about getting too much calcium from a pill emerged in several recent studies. Data from almost 24,000 people in the European Prospective Investigation into Cancer and Nutrition found that taking 2,000 mg of calcium or more per day seems to boost heart attack risk.

While the jury's still out on this link because of some concerns about the data, it's important to know that if your calcium intake is low, your body will "steal" calcium from your bones to get what it needs for other jobs like regulating blood pressure.

Still, don't overdo. The Institute of Medicine recommends that women younger than 51 and men younger than 71 get 1,000 mg a day *from food*, adding supplements if needed. Bump it up to 1,200 mg after those birthdays. Be sure you're also getting 600 IU of vitamin D daily if you're younger than 71; 800 IU after that because D helps you absorb calcium.

To decide whether or not you need a supplement, tally the calcium in your diet first. If you're getting two to three servings of dairy foods and at least one of leafy greens daily, you may be getting plenty. If not, add up to 500 mg of calcium a day.

 Daily calcium (along with enough vitamin D) could reduce your bone-fracture risk by an impressive 25%, report researchers from Australia's University of Western Sydney. The same combo—along with magnesium and other nutrients in dairy foods—may cut your risk for type 2 diabetes 15% by helping you stay sensitive to insulin, the hormone that tells cells to sip blood sugar, say Tufts University researchers.

MEN: THINK TWICE ABOUT FISH OIL

Incorporating at least 12 ounces of fish into your diet per week (4 oz, 3X per week) is a great way to optimize omega-3 fatty acid intake, and replaces less desirable protein sources like red meat (which are high in saturated fat). Don't love seafood? Adding walnuts, ground flaxseed or chia seeds, and lots of leafy greens will help you meet your needs. Talk to your doctor about a DHA/EPA supplement if you're concerned about getting enough."

—**JACLYN LONDON**, MS, RD, NUTRITION DIRECTOR, GOOD HOUSEKEEPING INSTITUTE

But there's a "but." In new research from the Fred Hutchinson Cancer Center in Seattle, men who ate a lot of fatty fish and men who took high-potency fish oil capsules turned out to be at higher risk for aggressive prostate cancer. So if you're a man, especially if you have a family history of prostate cancer, discuss this supplement with your doctor before taking it.

WHY IT HELPS → Years of research show that omega-3s—found in fatty fish like salmon as well as in flaxseed, walnuts, and some greens—can reduce anxiety, lower odds for Alzheimer's and other memory problems, and even help protect against type 2 diabetes. That's why fish oil capsules and other supplements that contain omega-3s are international bestsellers, with sales set to exceed $34 billion by 2016. They just may not be right for everybody.

· GOOD · HOUSEKEEPING
QUALITY TESTED
Since ★ 1909
LIMITED WARRANTY · ghseal.com for details

"If you're low in iron, cooking in a cast iron pan is a great way to get some into you're your diet. Every time you cook in it, a little bit will leach into your food."

—**SHARON FRANKE**, DIRECTOR, GOOD HOUSEKEEPING KITCHEN APPLIANCES AND TECHNOLOGY LAB

10-SECOND SOLUTIONS

COQ10 AND CHOLESTEROL

Coenzyme Q10 is a vitamin-like substance that helps your cells create energy. But cholesterol-lowering statin drugs (such as Lipitor) block the formation of CoQ10. This can lead to muscle cramps, memory impairment, and other complications.

—JOSEPH MAROON, MD, PROFESSOR OF NEUROSURGERY AT THE UNIVERSITY OF PITTSBURGH AND AUTHOR OF *THE LONGEVITY FACTOR*

If you're taking a statin, you should be taking 100 mg of CoQ10. If not, ask your doctor why.

—JOHN PAN, MD, FOUNDER OF THE GEORGE WASHINGTON UNIVERSITY CENTER FOR INTEGRATIVE MEDICINE

DO YOU NEED A MULTI WITH IRON?

The *only* people who need a multivitamin with iron are women in their menstruating years. Monthly menstruation can reduce iron stores, so their daily requirement from food and supplements is 18 mg (27 mg daily during pregnancy). Who should *not* take a multi with iron: postmenopausal women and men of any age. Your needs are much lower (8 mg daily) and far easier to meet with food. Too much iron ups your risk for heart disease and even liver damage.

Don't take extra unless you're diagnosed with anemia. Don't self-diagnose. It's easy to ask your doctor for a blood test to check your levels and get advice on supplementing.

—DARIUSH MOZAFFARIAN, MD, ASSOCIATE PROFESSOR OF MEDICINE, HARVARD SCHOOL OF PUBLIC HEALTH

WHEN TO TAKE PROBIOTICS

If you've been taking an antibiotic and struggling with diarrhea as a result, add a probiotic. It helps replace the good bacteria that got wiped out when the drug attacked the bad bugs (antibiotics can't tell good from bad). Look for probiotics containing *Lactobacillus* strains such as *L. rhamnosus* or *L. casei*. Both have been well studied and found to help. Probiotics that contain live strains in spore form have a better chance of getting into your gut. Check labels.

—MICHAEL F. ROIZEN, MD, CHIEF WELLNESS OFFICER AT THE CLEVELAND CLINIC AND CO-AUTHOR OF *YOU: THE OWNER'S MANUAL*

WHY IT HELPS → Your digestive system uses good bacteria (probiotics) to convert food into nutrients and keep your GI tract healthy. In some studies, these beneficial "bugs" also lower the risk of irritable bowel syndrome, vaginal yeast infections, and even depression. Good bacteria can bolster immunity, too, and may help control weight.

Normally, eating yogurt with live active cultures can help keep your own personal herd of good bugs going strong. So can munching the fibers that probiotics thrive on, found in bananas, onions, garlic, leeks, asparagus, artichokes, and soybeans, as well as whole-wheat breads, crackers, and cereals. But it often takes more than this to counter the side effects of an antibiotic.

"Choose plain (preferably Greek—it's higher in protein) yogurt with at least five different cultures listed in the ingredients list. Eat plenty of veggies and fruit, and be mindful to load up on foods rich in prebiotic fibers, like bananas. Since it may often take more than this to counter the long-term GI side effects of antibiotics, taking probiotic supplements like Culturelle or Florastor may be recommended."

—JACLYN LONDON, MS, RD, GOOD HOUSEKEEPING NUTRITION DIRECTOR

FIVE VITAMINS NOT TO OVERDO

DO NOT OVERDO VITAMINS, ESPECIALLY THESE FIVE:

1 **VITAMIN A.** Taking large amounts (more than 1,500 micrograms daily) can trigger dizziness, nausea, headaches, and joint pain.

2 **VITAMIN B6.** Over time, high doses of one to six grams a day can cause temporary nerve damage and digestive upsets.

3 **VITAMIN C.** Men who regularly take 1,000 mg or more of C double their risk for kidney stones, according to a 2013 study from Sweden.

4 **VITAMIN D.** Big doses boost your risk for irregular heart rhythms and kidney stones. The safe daily limit is 4,000 IU, but few experts advise taking that much, even though many consider the current recommendations somewhat low (600 IU before age 71 and 800 IU after that).

5 **VITAMIN E.** Mega-doses of more than about 1,000 mg per day are linked to hemorrhagic strokes.

NOT EVERYONE SHOULD TAKE B12

If you take a multivitamin, ask your doctor for a vitamin B12 test before you take extra on your own. For most people, the amount of B12 in a multi is plenty. But there are exceptions. After age 50 a drop in stomach acid can hinder B12 absorption. You may also be short if you take metformin for diabetes or drugs for heartburn, such as omeprazole (Prilosec), lansoprazole (Prevacid), or famotidine (Pepcid).

In addition, some people just have a hard time absorbing B12. And others have food conflicts that limit their B12 intake—for instance, an allergy to dairy or shellfish, or an aversion to eating meat.

—MAX LANGHURST, A NATUROPATHIC SPECIALIST IN NEW YORK CITY

WHY IT HELPS → Vitamin B12 is most famous as an energizing nutrient that helps your body build red blood cells, nerves, and DNA. It also plays an important role in the complex system that protects your genes—mess-ups may increase risk for cancer. And it's needed for proper metabolism of homocysteine, which ups heart-disease risk if levels get too high.

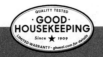

DO YOUR HOMEWORK

"From a regulatory perspective, dietary supplements are considered a food category. The US Food and Drug Administration does not require manufacturers and distributors to obtain approval before marketing dietary supplements, putting the onus on the firm to ensure the products it manufactures or distributes are safe and work as claimed. Therefore, not all nutritional supplements on the market today are manufactured using the rigorous practices used for prescription and over-the-counter drugs. Even though supplements are not regulated as drugs, they can have strong effects in the body and may interact with any other prescription or over-the-counter medications you are taking. Therefore, you should consult your physician on the type, dose, and brand name before taking any supplements. If your doctor won't specify a brand name, look for third-party certifications from NSF or USP, which ensure that the product's manufacturing practices meet or exceed the good manufacturing practices used by the pharmaceutical manufacturers and that the dosage of the vitamins and minerals is present at the amounts stated on the label."

—**BIRNUR ARAL**, PHD, DIRECTOR, GOOD HOUSEKEEPING HEALTH, BEAUTY AND ENVIRONMENTAL SCIENCES LAB

ANSWERS TO
SUPPLEMENT SMARTS

1 **FALSE.** Despite news about studies claiming that multi-vitamins offer no health benefits, the truth is that they do. Research shows that men who take a multi lower their prostate cancer risk, and people who take a multi can reduce risk for colon polyps by 20%. The right multi can also protect your vision and, for women of child-bearing age, help prevent birth defects in future babies. *See page 61.*

2 **C.** Yes, your skin produces vitamin D when sunlight hits it, but only if the rays are strong enough. And they're usually not if you live north of an imaginary line between San Francisco and Richmond, Virginia. Also, few foods contain enough vitamin D to deliver all you need. So aim for at least 600 IU a day from a supplement, 800 IU after age 70. Many D experts say 1,000 IU is even better. *See page 52.*

3 **B.** While your body uses and needs all three forms of good omega-3 fats, DHA—the most potent form—has a special affinity for your brain. In fact, your brain is largely made up of omega-3s, and 97% are DHA. You can get this "super fat" from cold-water fish like salmon and mackerel, and from omega-3

supplements such as fish oil capsules. *See page 53.*

4 **ALL THREE ARE CORRECT.** Don't take B12 on your own; many people get plenty from food and their multi. But if you're over 50, take heartburn drugs, or don't eat meat, you may need more B12 due to absorption problems or a dietary gap. *See page 58.*

5 **FALSE.** Be careful about popping high doses of C. In one Swedish study, taking 1,000 mg or more on a regular basis doubled the risk for kidney stones. The daily recommendation is 75 to 90 mg, though that's often considered too low. *See page 58.*

6 **A.** Probiotics are good bacteria in your intestinal tract that help digest food. They've been making headlines as researchers discover more and more probiotic benefits. Having a healthy mix inside you may help control weight, lower risk for depression, promote healthy digestion, and bolster immunity. But so far, research suggests that these supplements are most useful if you have diarrhea due to antibiotics. *See page 57.*

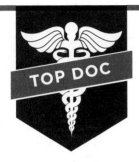

TOP DOC

KEEP THIS SMART SUPPLEMENT ADVICE IN MIND

When it comes to supplements, top docs don't under- or overdo. Use these five reminders to turn their good advice into a smart supplement strategy for you:

1 A MULTIVITAMIN'S STILL A WORTHWHILE INSURANCE POLICY. Top preventive medicine docs say there are enough benefits to warrant continuing to take one to lower risk for colon polyps, vision problems, prostate cancer, and probably more.

2 TOP DOCS AND NUTRITION EXPERTS RECOMMEND OMEGA-3S AND A LITTLE CALCIUM, TOO. Talk with your own physician about the omega-3 dose that's right for you, especially if you're a man. And use calcium supplements when your daily intake from leafy greens and dairy foods isn't quite high enough.

3 ADD VITAMIN D. Aim for 600 to 1,000 IU of D per day. If you take a multi and a calcium supplement that contains D (many do because D helps bones absorb calcium), you may already get that much. If not, add a separate vitamin D supplement to make up the difference. Very few people get enough D from food and/or sun exposure.

4 TALK WITH YOUR DOC FIRST ABOUT TAKING OTHER INDIVIDUAL NUTRIENTS. You *may* need extra B12 or CoQ10. But check in with your MD anyway. Every top doc wants you to follow the same rule they do: "Don't take anything you don't need."

5 SAY NO TO HIGH DOSES. Whether it's vitamin A, B6, C, D, E, or something else, taking mega-doses can do harm instead of good. Don't risk it.

SLEEP & ENERGY SECRETS

RECENT POLL FOUND THAT 38% OF WORKING ADULTS (INCLUDING YOU?) FEEL FATIGUED MOST DAYS OF THE WEEK. As you'll discover in this chapter, physicians have discovered plenty of ways to help their patients optimize their get-up-and-go.

AMONG THEIR ADVICE:

CATCH UP ON WEEKENDS. If you average 7.5 hours of shut-eye per night on weekends, that's enough to erase at least some sleep debt, research shows.

ENERGIZE WITH EXERCISE. Two out of three docs say they use physical activity to recharge. They recommend the same strategy to their patients.

NAP. These days, even physicians-in-training are urged to power-nap during downtime in order to boost alertness. A smart napping strategy can work for you, too.

DRINK COFFEE STRATEGICALLY. An average of two cups a day is enough to stay awake but not enough to interfere with a good night's sleep.

Ahead, you'll find out what doctors recommend to fall asleep fast, get enough deep sleep to recharge mind and body, wake up feeling refreshed, and then stay sharp and alert throughout very long days. In their energy kits: everything from smart snacks to aromatherapy.

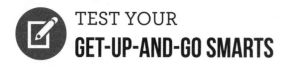

TEST YOUR
GET-UP-AND-GO SMARTS

Deeper sleep tonight. More energy tomorrow. Everyone wants both—along with better health, happier moods, and more productive days. Test your knowledge about the surprising strategies that time-pressed docs rely on, and that are often as easy as they are effective. Then dig in to the chapter for how-tos and details.

1 You didn't sleep well last night and need a surefire way to stay alert today, so you:

a. Drink a huge mug of coffee first thing, and chug a second just in case.

b. Have an energy bar or bran-nut muffin along with a large cup of Joe.

c. Sip one caffeinated drink slowly throughout the morning and into the afternoon.

2 Which drug-free energy booster is proven to lift deep fatigue in business travelers, older adults, cancer survivors, and people who simply feel tired all the time?

a. An ice-cold, fruit-filled smoothie

b. A short, relaxed walk

c. Green tea

3 Need an afternoon nap? You'll feel most refreshed if you sleep for:

a. 14 minutes

b. 26 minutes

c. 61 minutes

4 Thanks to busy schedules, hours of homework, and bedroom electronics, plenty of school kids skimp on sleep these days. They need this much:

a. Eleven hours during elementary school, 9.25 hours after that

b. Nine hours for elementary schoolers, eight hours for tweens and teens

c. Eight solid hours for all school-age kids

5 Why are cold cereal and hot oatmeal such good sleepy-time snacks?

a. They're comfort foods that remind you of childhood.

b. They're easy to digest.

c. They contain nutrients that tilt your body chemistry toward slumber.

6 Inhaling the sweet scent of jasmine can help you:

a. Fall asleep faster

b. Feel alert and on your game

c. Wake up earlier

FIND THE ANSWERS ON PAGE 76!

WAKE UP WITH NATURAL LIGHT

Here's one way I recharge my internal battery daily: I make sure I get high-quality sleep at night. To do this, I dim the lights one hour before bedtime and sleep in a pitch-black room. When I wake up in the morning, I make sure I get some sunshine right away. I'll work near a window or in the garden or take a walk outside. Bright morning light turns off your brain's secretion of sleep-inducing melatonin *and* stimulates the production of serotonin, which helps you feel energized.

—**JOEL FUHRMAN**, MD, RESEARCH DIRECTOR OF THE NUTRITIONAL RESEARCH FOUNDATION IN FLEMINGTON, NEW JERSEY, AND AUTHOR OF *THE END OF HEART DISEASE*, AMONG OTHER BOOKS

WHY IT WORKS → Sunset's natural dimming triggers the release of sleep-inducing melatonin a few hours before sleep—or it would if you weren't surrounded by bright indoor lights, especially the blue-tinged light waves from TVs, computer screens, smartphones, and other electronics, which can be stimulating. Bright lights stall melatonin's release, play havoc with your natural sleep rhythms, and, over time, may even affect your health and longevity.

Left-on artificial light also causes trouble after you're asleep, too, because light can pass through your eyelids and mess with your melatonin. That's why Fuhrman sleeps in a pitch-black bedroom. Some people even cover lit clocks. And some electronics have tools to reduce brightness of screens at night.

By contrast, light exposure during the day is energizing. Morning light sends a wake-up call along nerve pathways from your eyes to your internal clock. And researchers say that a dose of sunshine at midday boosts alertness and mood, too.

SIP, DON'T GULP, CAFFEINE

I have a reputation for drinking coffee all day long—but it's really the same cup. I just sip it, not gulp it. When it gets cold, I pretend it's iced coffee. Caffeine blocks adenosine, a sleep-inducing brain chemical that builds up during the day. But if you drink all your coffee first thing in the morning, its effects wear off around siesta time, just when you need it most.

However, if you give yourself small, regular doses of caffeine—that is, take spread-out sips rather than chugging it all at once—you can wipe out the fatigue that often creeps in later on. Just stop around midafternoon. Drinking coffee too late in the day can mess up your sleep that night.

—JAMES K. WYATT, PHD, DIRECTOR OF THE SECTION OF SLEEP DISORDERS AND SLEEP-WAKE RESEARCH AT RUSH UNIVERSITY MEDICAL CENTER, CHICAGO

WHY IT WORKS → If you're short on sleep or working a crazy schedule, nursing a cup of coffee through the morning can also counteract daytime fatigue and sleepiness. This became clear when researchers simulated the long, sleep-deprived days of medical residents and first responders, like firefighters and emergency crews. In a month-long study conducted at the Brigham and Women's Hospital in Boston, they kept volunteers awake for more than 28 hours at a stretch, then let them sleep about 14 hours. Afterward, they tested small, frequent doses of caffeine.

The result? Those who got a pill every hour containing the amount of caffeine in about two ounces of coffee scored better on mental tests than those who got a fake pill.

SKIP COUNTING SHEEP

When my brain's on overload, I use progressive relaxation to coax myself to sleep. I visualize each part of my body and imagine it completely at rest, starting at my toes. Then I move upward one muscle group at a time until I reach the crown of the head. This almost always makes me doze off.

—CARL BAZIL, MD, DIRECTOR OF THE DIVISION OF SLEEP AND EPILEPSY IN THE DEPARTMENT OF NEUROLOGY AT COLUMBIA UNIVERSITY IN NEW YORK CITY

 → While this may seem like a "no big deal" exercise, researchers beg to differ. There's good evidence that this low-tech, free, do-anywhere technique is excellent at bringing on sleep when you're tense because it gradually de-stresses your whole body.

IT ALSO HELPS OTHER STRESS-RELATED ISSUES, INCLUDING:

▶ **HIGH BLOOD PRESSURE.** Doing progressive muscle relaxation twice daily for three months can reduce your systolic pressure (the top number). In studies, it lowered it by about five points. That's a lot.

▶ **FREQUENT TENSION HEADACHES.** In Swiss research, relaxation training worked better than acupuncture or exercise for preventing tension headaches.

▶ **RADIATION FATIGUE.** When people get radiation treatments for cancer, just 15 to 20 minutes of daily progressive relaxation significantly eases that wiped-out feeling.

TAKE A PERFECT NAP

A friend of mine with a new baby was getting up a lot at night and felt zonked during the day. She tried taking naps, but they weren't helping. Turns out she was setting her alarm for 60 minutes. She didn't know that an average sleep cycle is 90 minutes, so she was waking up when her body was in the deepest stages of sleep.

No wonder she felt groggy, not rested! For a quick pick-me-up, she should take a 20-minute nap, which I told her. British researchers say that a 20-minute afternoon snooze boosts energy more than two cups of coffee.

But when she's trying to catch up after a particularly sleepless night with the baby, a 90-minute nap is better. It will get her through an entire sleep cycle and she'll wake up refreshed.

—W. CHRISTOPHER WINTER, MD, MEDICAL DIRECTOR OF CHARLOTTESVILLE NEUROLOGY AND SLEEP MEDICINE IN VIRGINIA AND SLEEP SPECIALIST FOR NUMEROUS PROFESSIONAL SPORTS ORGANIZATIONS

WHY IT WORKS → Short is often sweet when it comes to daytime sleep. In a NASA-funded study of long-haul airline pilots, those who got a 26-minute nap kicked up their performance by 34%. In other research, nappers who splashed their faces with cold water afterward felt the most awake. Don't want to disturb your hair or makeup? After a nap, wash your hands in cold water and pat some on the back of your neck.

"Hungry before bed? Skip chocolate, peppermint, tomatoes/tomato sauce, and orange juice—all of which can keep you awake if you're prone to acid reflux. Fatty foods (anything fried, tons of cheese and nuts, or meat) will also get in the way of your sleep cycle since they take significantly longer to digest and absorb."

—JACLYN LONDON, MS, RD, GOOD HOUSEKEEPING NUTRITION DIRECTOR

SNIFF JASMINE
FOR AN ENERGY LIFT

Could the heady scent of jasmine up your game? Maybe. Sniffing jasmine helped amateur bowlers improve their scores by an impressive 26%, according to small studies at Chicago's Smell and Taste Treatment and Research Foundation. It also enhanced the batting of six Major League Baseball players, said the players *and* their batting coaches.

My sons play basketball and ice hockey. When I told them about smelling jasmine boosting these athletic performances, they tested it themselves, dabbing jasmine extract on their wristbands. They also thought it helped.

—ALAN R. HIRSCH, MD, FACP, NEUROLOGICAL DIRECTOR OF THE SMELL AND TASTE TREATMENT AND RESEARCH FOUNDATION IN CHICAGO, AND SENIOR ATTENDING PHYSICIAN AT MERCY HOSPITAL AND MEDICAL CENTER

WHY IT WORKS → "Jasmine seems to improve hand-eye coordination by reducing anxiety and/or increasing alertness," says Hirsch. "At the bowling alley, it may also help simply by covering up the mixed smells of bowling shoes, pizza, and beer! Another possibility: When you're pushing your body hard, a pleasing scent could distract you from muscle fatigue."

The scent of jasmine could improve precise hand-eye coordination in areas besides sports, such as surgery, musical performance, and physical therapy. Other scents have benefits, too. Hirsch has found that regularly sniffing peppermint, banana, and/or green apple scents can aid weight loss by stimulating a feeling of fullness and reducing overeating. Peppermint also boosts alertness, and green apple eases migraine pain in people who enjoy its sharp, tart smell.

EIGHT "GET SLEEPY" FOODS

A plate makeover can help you catch more high-quality ZZZs. In fact, eating the right foods at the right time may help you fall asleep *faster* as well as sleep better. Our doctor-recommended "get ready for sleep" list and why each one works:

1 ALMONDS. "They're a winner. Almonds contain magnesium, which promotes both sleep and muscle relaxation. And they supply protein, which helps keep your blood sugar stable while you're sleeping," says Jacob Teitelbaum, MD, creator of the popular free app Cures A–Z and author of *From Fatigued to Fantastic!*

2 CEREAL. A small serving of whole-grain, low-sugar cereal with low-fat milk tilts your body chemistry toward sleep. "Foods rich in complex carbohydrates increase the availability of tryptophan in the bloodstream, which may increase its sleep-inducing effects," says Saundra Dalton-Smith, MD, Alabama internist, author, and founder of IChooseMyBestLife.com.

3 DAIRY FOODS. While yogurt, milk, and cheese contain some tryptophan, it's their abundant sleep-inducing calcium that may send you off to dreamland. "Calcium is effective in stress reduction and stabilizing nerves, including the brain's," says Dalton-Smith.

4 EDAMAME (SNACK-READY SOY BEANS). For menopausal women, "the natural estrogen-like compounds found in soy foods may be beneficial in countering the hot flashes that so often disturb sleep," says Dalton-Smith.

5 HARDBOILED EGGS. Having a high-protein egg as a pre-bedtime snack may help you stay asleep, unlike blood sugar-spiking cookies or ice cream. "The problem with the refined carbs in sweets is that they can put you on a sugar roller-coaster and drop your blood sugar while you're sleeping, making you wake at 2 or 3 a.m.," says Teitelbaum.

6 HERBAL OR GREEN TEA. "Chamomile tea is a safe, helpful sleep aid. And green tea contains theanine, which helps promote sleep. Just be sure it's decaf green tea!" says Teitelbaum.

7 MISO SOUP. Keeping some instant miso soup on hand—the comforting broth that's a staple in Japanese restaurants—could be just the thing when you can't fall asleep. Why? Miso contains amino acids, which appear to boost the production of melatonin, the natural hormone that helps induce yawns, according to Stella Metsovas, CN, nutritionist in Laguna Beach, California.

8 OATMEAL. Could a bowl of hot oatmeal help you get more rest? "Oatmeal is warm, soft, soothing, easy to prepare, and nourishing. It's also rich in calcium, magnesium, phosphorus, silicon, and potassium—practically a 'who's who' of the nutrients that support sleep," says Stephan Dorlandt, CN, nutritionist based in Southern California.

TRY THIS
PRE-BED SNACK

"Dried cherries + pistachios. Pistachios have a winning sleep-inducing combination of protein, vitamin B6, and magnesium, and research has shown that cherries can help improve melatonin production. Just don't exceed a 1-ounce portion of nuts (about 160 calories) and 1 cup of cherries, since anything too high in calories can have the reverse effect of keeping you awake."

—**JACLYN LONDON**, MS, RD, GOOD HOUSEKEEPING NUTRITION DIRECTOR

10-SECOND SOLUTIONS

DOUBLE A NAP'S ENERGY REWARDS

Try sipping a cup of coffee just before a 20-minute nap. By the time the caffeine kicks in, it will be time to wake up and you'll feel doubly refreshed and alert, say researchers from Britain's Loughborough University.

HOW FIRM SHOULD A MATTRESS BE?

Medium-firm, report researchers at Oklahoma State University. Medium-firm support tested best at improving sleep comfort and quality, and reducing back and shoulder pain.

UPGRADE YOUR PILLOWS

Once a year I take stock of my bedding. That almost always means changing my pillows so they better support my head and neck. I prefer soft foam ones but they don't last that long. I also make sure my mattress isn't breaking down. A good-quality new one every five to eight years can give you the best sleep of your life.

—**MICHAEL BREUS**, PHD, AUTHOR OF *THE POWER OF WHEN: DISCOVER YOUR CHRONOTYPE—AND THE BEST TIME TO EAT LUNCH, ASK FOR A RAISE, HAVE SEX, WRITE A NOVEL, TAKE YOUR MEDS, AND MORE*

TELL YOUR BRAIN, "GO TO SLEEP"

When I take a nap, I use a sound machine that creates "pink noise"—a blend of high- and low-frequency sounds. It blocks out any nearby noise and helps me relax. But maybe even more important, it's like an auditory mantra for relaxation and rest. The sound it makes is so unusual that whenever I hear it, it says to my brain, "Time to sleep." Though heaven help me if I'm ever driving down the road and hear that sound!

I also use a very soft pillow spritzed with a little sleep-promoting lavender scent and a cozy blanket that is soft as kitten fur. It's all about having sounds, sensations, and aromas that say, "This is when we relax and go to sleep."

—**W. CHRISTOPHER WINTER**, MD, MEDICAL DIRECTOR OF CHARLOTTESVILLE NEUROLOGY AND SLEEP MEDICINE IN VIRGINIA AND SLEEP SPECIALIST FOR NUMEROUS PROFESSIONAL SPORTS ORGANIZATIONS

 Creating your own fall-asleep routine—whether for naps or at night—is a widely recommended strategy that works for kids and adults. In a study at Philadelphia's St. Joseph's University, mothers who established consistent bedtime routines for their infants and toddlers said their kids slept better and woke up less during the night. Bedtime routines that include special cues help adults sleep better, too, says the National Sleep Foundation. Dimming the lights, doing gentle stretching, taking a warm shower, brushing your teeth, snuggling into bed with a good book or soothing music—routinely doing some or all of these can quickly open the door to dreamland.

ENFORCE BEDTIMES FOR KIDS

My daughter has had a set bedtime since she was very young to ensure she gets enough sleep. She's a teenager now, but we still continue that practice. She says she was one of the only kids in high school who got at least eight hours a night, and most nights she got nine.

Our routine for her included a shower or bath, brushing her teeth, and then always reading a book. When she was very young, every single night was *Goodnight Moon!* As she got older, we switched to chapter books like *Charlie and the Chocolate Factory*. Eventually, my husband read the entire Harry Potter series to her.

She continues to read every night at bedtime. And of course, there are no TVs or electronics in her bedroom!

—**JODI A. MINDELL**, PHD, ASSOCIATE DIRECTOR OF THE SLEEP CENTER AT THE CHILDREN'S HOSPITAL OF PHILADELPHIA AND AUTHOR OF *SLEEPING THROUGH THE NIGHT: HOW INFANTS, TODDLERS, AND THEIR PARENTS CAN GET A GOOD NIGHT'S SLEEP*

WHY IT WORKS → Whether they're toddlers or teens, studies show that kids in general don't get the sleep they need, up to several hours a night. Sufficient sleep—roughly 12 to 15 hours a day for preschoolers, 11 hours for elementary-age kids, and 9.25 hours for middle schoolers and teens—helps kids perform better in school. But skimping on sleep increases their risks for weight gain, obesity, and even premature high blood pressure and blood sugar problems. Tuck 'em in!

From the beginning, ensure that your child has an early bedtime and a consistent bedtime routine, emphasizes Mindell. "A nightly bedtime routine is a way to wind down and tell your brain, 'It's time to go to bed.'"

SHORT, EASY EXERCISE PERKS

Dragging through your day? A 20-minute stroll—and we do mean stroll, not a speed walk—will pick you up without tiring you out. This kind of exercising for energy helps all sorts of people who are dealing with deep fatigue.

 SOME EXAMPLES:

▶ **COUCH POTATOES GET A BUZZ.** University of Georgia scientists tested mild exercise on a group of sedentary people who said they always felt tired. The volunteers did either low- or moderate-intensity workouts on exercise bikes three times a week for six weeks. The surprising result: The low-intensity group got the biggest energy lift: a 65% drop in fatigue. The moderate-intensity exercisers got only a 49% drop—good, but less. The researchers suspect the somewhat tougher routine tired them a bit.

▶ **BUSINESS TRAVELERS RECOVER THEIR ZING.** In a small study, business travelers who worked out on the road did 61% better on mental tests than their sedentary colleagues.

▶ **OLDER ADULTS FEEL MORE ALERT.** Almost 40% of people aged 65 and up who did gentle yoga or chair-based exercises for eight weeks felt more energetic, say researchers at New York City's Hospital for Special Surgery.

▶ **PEOPLE WITH DEEP FATIGUE RALLY.** "Lite" exercise has been shown to ease fatigue in survivors of cancer and heart attacks, and people with chronic fatigue syndrome. Going through any of these? Ask your doctor about special routines that can help.

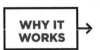 Easygoing exercise seems to chase away fatigue by increasing three energizing brain chemicals: dopamine, norepinephrine, and serotonin. It also boosts circulation, which brings more energizing oxygen to your brain and muscles, and may improve sleep, too.

ANSWERS TO
GET-UP-AND-GO SMARTS

1 **C.** Research from Chicago's Rush University Medical Center shows that small sip-size "doses" of caffeine spread out over several hours energize you better for the long haul than one big hit in the morning. The reason: Caffeine blocks a brain chemical that makes you feel drowsy, so as caffeine wears off, the desire to nod off gets stronger. Taking a few regular sips every hour counteracts this effect. *See page 66.*

2 **B.** It sounds paradoxical, but physical activity is emerging as the solution for all sorts of fatigue (not just normal sloth!). To make it work, exercise regularly but not too vigorously—don't push so hard that you feel exhausted. In one study, people with garden-variety fatigue who got light, consistent exercise perked up more than those who worked out more intensely. *See page 75.*

3 **B.** Set your alarm to ring in 26 minutes. Heavy sleepers may think such a short nap couldn't possibly be enough, but sleep studies confirm that keeping naps short and sweet is effective. What about the classic one-hour nap? Experts say it'll leave you feeling groggy because your brain will be in the middle of a longer, deeper sleep cycle when your alarm goes off. *See page 68.*

4 **A.** Yup, kids and teens need lots of sleep. But many are running deficits ranging from one to even six hours—a gap that can harm school performance and contribute to weight gain. Help the kids in your life by enforcing bedtimes and helping them establish a soothing sleep routine, like a warm bath or shower and some quiet reading. Nix electronics at least 30 minutes before they're getting ready to turn in. *See page 74.*

5 **C.** The complex carbohydrates in whole grains increase the availability of snooze-inducing compounds in your body. And the minerals in whole grains—such as calcium, magnesium, phosphorus, silicon, and potassium—all support sound sleep. *See page 70.*

6 **B.** Sniffing jasmine increased performance and alertness in athletes as diverse as NBA players and amateur bowlers in fascinating tests done by Chicago's Smell and Taste Treatment and Research Foundation. Don't like jasmine? Try peppermint; it has similar energy-enhancing effects. *See page 69.*

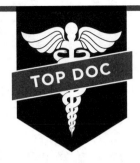

REMEMBER THESE FIVE ENERGIZING SLEEP STRATEGIES

Follow these steps to turn the solutions from top docs into an easy blueprint for sound sleep tonight, high energy tomorrow:

1 **BE SMART ABOUT CAFFEINE.** Whether you get yours from a fancy coffee shop, a homemade cup of tea, or a can of cola, knowing how to use caffeine to stay alert (without staying up half the night) is crucial. The trick: Make your morning cup last for several hours, and don't sip it late in the afternoon or evening; caffeine blocks a brain chemical that makes you fall asleep . . . leading to more fatigue tomorrow.

2 **MAKE IT EASY FOR YOUR BODY AND BRAIN TO FALL ASLEEP.** Top docs recommend creating soothing bedtime routines and keeping your bedroom cool, dark, and quiet—all steps proven to welcome sleep. Then snap open your shades in the morning. Exposure to morning light resets your body clock and revs up your system for a high-energy day.

3 **GET COMFY.** The right bedding doesn't have to cost a fortune, but it should feel like a million bucks to you. Top docs recommend giving your pillows and mattress an annual checkup for soothing comfort and supportive rest.

4 **LIFT FATIGUE WITH EASY EXERCISE.** Light activity relieves fatigue whether you're jet-lagged, regrouping from cancer treatment, recovering from a heart attack, or just feel wiped-out. Movement relieves stress, increases circulation, and helps you get a better night's sleep.

5 **TAKE KIDS' SLEEP NEEDS SERIOUSLY.** They need your help to get enough shut-eye. Top docs recommend enforcing bedtimes, and not just for small fry. Tweens and teens need to turn in on time, too. Forbid using electronics at bedtime and overnight. Lack of sleep boosts kids' risk of weight and blood pressure problems.

CHAPTER 5

ALTERNATIVE MEDICINE ADVICE

HERE'S A SURPRISE: Doctors and nurses are way more likely to use complementary therapies—from herbs and meditation to self-hypnosis, massage, yoga, and acupuncture—than the rest of us are, say researchers from the University of Minnesota and Allina Hospitals and Clinics in Minneapolis, who polled 1,280 healthcare practitioners about their use of alternative medicine. By comparison, only 63% of Americans have tried or use it.

So much for that image of the buttoned-up doc who sticks with conservative care. Top docs today know that alternative and complementary therapies boost well-being, frequently help conventional treatments work better, and often offer relief for everything from cold symptoms to sleep issues to stress.

Doctors' acceptance of alternative medicine is a win-win for them and their patients, believes Lori Knutson, RN, of Allina Hospitals and Clinics. "It creates an opening on both sides to optimize health for the whole person," she says. Coming up: alternative and complementary remedies that top physicians use themselves and recommend their patients consider, too.

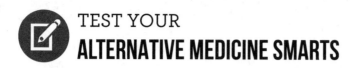

TEST YOUR
ALTERNATIVE MEDICINE SMARTS

"Complementary" and conventional medicine may sometimes seem worlds apart, but top docs recommend crossing the divide more frequently than the rest of us realize. Are you savvy about what kinds of nontraditional medicine make a real health difference? Test your knowledge with this quiz, then check out which remedies top docs endorse for themselves, their families, and their patients.

1 Meditation eases stress and is known to improve health. To tap some of its benefits, simply sit quietly once a day and focus on rhythmic breathing for:

a. 1 hour

b. 30 minutes

c. 5 minutes

2 Elderberry syrup sounds like a dessert topping, but it's actually a research-proven way to relieve:

a. Flu

b. Constipation

c. Allergies

3 Acupuncture—the ancient Chinese healing art that involves sliding fine needles into precise points on the body—can help your health by:

a. Easing specific conditions, such as pain, headaches, digestive disorders, or anxiety

b. Enhancing well-being, even if you're not sick

c. Both

d. Neither

4 Show your next headache who's boss by gently pressing here:

a. On your chin

b. Just below the middle of each eyebrow

c. On your wrist an inch away from your palm

5 Skin-friendly botanicals that can soothe irritated skin include:

a. Calendula and aloe

b. Dandelion and valerian

c. Cat's claw and gingko

6 One way to get a fast massage for stiff shoulders or an aching back is to:

a. Go to a mall with one of those walk-in massage-chain salons.

b. Spring for an electric massage chair pad.

c. Lie down on a tennis ball.

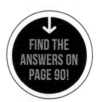

FIND THE ANSWERS ON PAGE 90!

GET NEEDLED ROUTINELY

I regularly schedule acupuncture appointments for myself. I find that it reduces both stress and physical pain, two things that deplete your body of energy.

—LISA AIRAN, MD, AESTHETIC DERMATOLOGIST IN NEW YORK CITY AND FORMER NATIONAL INSTITUTES OF HEALTH FELLOW

These doctors aren't alone. Many people turn to acupuncture for regular tune-ups that enhance well-being. This ancient healing technique involves inserting sterile, hair-thin needles at precise points on the body to unblock energy or qi (pronounced *chee*). Traditional practitioners sometimes twirl or heat the needles, but today's high-tech acupuncture may also use laser beams, sound waves, and mild electric current to stimulate qi.

Finally, research shows that acupuncture can ease a stunning variety of health conditions, from hay fever and high blood pressure to digestive disorders, insomnia, asthma, anxiety, depression, sinus infections, labor pain, and even infertility. It can also relieve many types of chronic pain, including headaches, joint aches, and some cancer pain.

 Science suggests that acupuncture triggers the release of pain-relieving compounds called opioid peptides in the brain and spinal cord. Somehow, the process also seems to make the brain "smarter" about pain by increasing the number of cell receptors that mute pain signals.

ASK ONE SIMPLE QUESTION

Throughout my day, I try to ask myself this simple question: What do I really need in this moment that is in my best interest? Nourishing food? A big stretch? A hug? A walk? If I take the time to listen to my body, listen to my heart, I am more likely to make good decisions for myself rather than impulsively reaching for the ice cream, skipping meals, going to bed too late, or watching TV instead of going for a walk. This question helps me pause and remember what is important to me so I can respond thoughtfully. Instead of living out of habit, I get to be in charge of my life.

—SUSAN B. LORD, MD, INTEGRATIVE PHYSICIAN PRACTICING IN HOUSATONIC, MASSACHUSETTS, AND EXECUTIVE DIRECTOR OF THE CENTER FOR PEACE THROUGH CULTURE

WHY IT WORKS → Research suggests that people who learn mindfulness techniques—such as having regular Q&As with their body or doing meditation (see "Take Out Your Mental Garbage," later in this chapter)—have happier relationships, make healthier food choices, feel less stressed out, and are better at managing chronic conditions like diabetes.

QUALITY TESTED
·GOOD·
HOUSEKEEPING
Since ★ 1909
LIMITED WARRANTY · ghseal.com for details

"Considering that homeopathic remedies are not regulated by the FDA and their safety and efficacy haven't been always proven, our advice to consumers is to consult their physicians before self-treating with a homeopathic remedy."

—BIRNUR ARAL, PHD, DIRECTOR, GOOD HOUSEKEEPING HEALTH, BEAUTY AND ENVIRONMENTAL SCIENCES LAB

KEEP A MASSAGE THERAPIST IN YOUR POCKET

Massage feels great . . . but if you don't have the time, money, or opportunity to indulge in one, you don't have to miss out. Self-massage works, too. I carry a tennis ball in my pocket to massage myself. Here's how: To massage your back and shoulders with a tennis ball, lie on your back on the floor with a tennis ball under you at a sore spot. Roll a little on the ball to zero in on the most tender area, then stop and relax for a few minutes. Move it to other achy spots and repeat.

As basic as it may seem, self-massage can be very effective. Self-massage eased knee pain in people with osteoarthritis in a 2013 study at the Holos University Graduate Seminary in Missouri. And in recent research by my team, a combination of massage therapy and self-massage techniques significantly reduced the aches of people with painful rheumatoid arthritis in their shoulders. It also improved their grip strength and the flexibility in their wrists, elbows, and shoulder joints.

I totally recommend getting a daily dose of touch, whether it's massage or self-massage. Focus especially on body parts that tend to "store" stress, such as your neck, shoulders, and back. Yoga works like massage when you press your hands, feet, legs, and/or arms into your mat. I do a 20-minute yoga routine every day that has these kinds of effects. So do movement classes that include lots of hands-on instruction, such as Pilates or even ballroom dancing.

—TIFFANY FIELD, PHD, DIRECTOR OF THE TOUCH RESEARCH INSTITUTE IN THE DEPARTMENT OF PEDIATRICS, UNIVERSITY OF MIAMI SCHOOL OF MEDICINE, FLORIDA

WHY IT WORKS → When a joint hurts, the muscles surrounding it become tense and less flexible, creating stiffness and making movement hurt. Massage with moderate pressure de-tenses stiff muscles and makes the joint area—and you—feel better.

TAKE OUT YOUR MENTAL GARBAGE

I recommend meditation to all my patients. Your thoughts, feelings, and beliefs about yourself are like a blueprint for your health and happiness. The science is clear: Negative, critical thoughts and worrying over time make us more susceptible to illness. Think of meditation as "taking out the garbage" in your life, mind, and body. Meditation is a powerful tool of transformation—a way to let go of negative thoughts and create stillness and peace inside you. Over time, you'll become more internally quiet, and this inner stillness begins to inform how you live your life. There will always be challenges, often difficult ones, but you can develop resilience through meditation.

—**SUSAN B. LORD**, MD, INTEGRATIVE PHYSICIAN PRACTICING IN HOUSATONIC, MASSACHUSETTS, AND EXECUTIVE DIRECTOR OF THE CENTER FOR PEACE THROUGH CULTURE

Here's a simple way to start practicing meditation that takes just five minutes. Sit in a comfortable, relaxed position; close your eyes; and focus on one thing. It could be repeating a calming word like *peace* or *love* (or, yes, *om*), or allowing your belly to be soft and relaxed, or putting your attention on your breath. Whenever your mind wanders (and it will), gently bring it back to your chosen focus. Do this every day for a few minutes, gradually increasing the time to 10 or 20 minutes. In time, you will develop the ability to stay focused, and your mind will wander less and less, which will translate into living more calmly. In other words, there will be less mental garbage in your life.

WHY IT WORKS → "We all have negative thoughts at times," says Lord, "but if negativity becomes a way of life, you start living in a perpetual state of stress that affects the nervous system, causing inflammation and setting the stage for disease." Relaxing periodically throughout the day builds resilience and a more positive outlook so you're happier and healthier.

PRESS TO CANCEL PAIN

Here's a great remedy I use myself for headaches: Take your thumbs and place them under your brows, just above the middle of your eye socket. Push in and up, like you're giving a thumbs-up. Then just hold for a few seconds. This pressure on the orbital nerve can make stress-related headaches disappear.

—SANJAY GUPTA, MD, CHIEF MEDICAL CORRESPONDENT FOR CNN AND ASSOCIATE CHIEF OF NEUROSURGERY AT ATLANTA'S GRADY MEMORIAL HOSPITAL

 → Acupressure is a hands-on, needle-free version of acupuncture that can hit the spot for relieving tension headaches and more. Like acupuncture, it is believed to work by improving the flow of energy along pathways called meridians in the body. In trained hands, it can be a sophisticated healing art—easing severe knee pain, back pain, labor pain, and fatigue, according to various studies. Simple forms of this traditional Chinese medicine work as do-it-yourself remedies.

HERE ARE TWO ACUPRESSURE TECHNIQUES TO TRY:

▶ **BOOST YOUR MOOD, BEAT INSOMNIA:** Use the thumb of your right hand to press on the crease where your palm meets your wrist—below your little finger. Hold for five minutes, then reverse hands and repeat.

▶ **EASE NECK AND HEAD PAIN:** Use your right index finger and thumb to squeeze the center of the web between the thumb and first finger on your left hand. Apply moderate pressure (it might ache a little) for about two minutes. Then do the same with the opposite hand.

10-SECOND SOLUTIONS

HONEY FOR COUGHS

In research done a few years ago at the Pennsylvania State University College of Medicine, the parents of 105 coughing kids aged 2 and up were asked to give their child a dose of honey or a cough syrup that tasted like honey. Parents whose kids got the real honey reported more improvement in their children's symptoms and a better night's sleep for all.

PS: Important! Don't give honey to kids younger than 12 months because it may contain spores that could cause infant botulism. After their first birthday, honey's no problem.

NATURAL SKIN SOOTHERS

Instead of a steroid cream, try a plant-based calendula cream for mild skin irritations. This herb is a natural mild antiseptic, ideal for minor burns and scrapes. Alternatively, keep an aloe plant on the window and break off a small piece when needed. The gel inside is a great remedy for mild burns and itchy, inflamed skin.

—**MICHAEL FINKELSTEIN**, MD, A PHYSICIAN BOARD-CERTIFIED IN INTEGRATIVE-HOLISTIC MEDICINE IN BEDFORD, NEW YORK, AND AUTHOR OF *SLOW MEDICINE: HOPE AND HEALING FOR CHRONIC ILLNESS*

SIP THREE HEALING HERBAL TEAS

Thousands of years before herbs came in capsules, there was tea. Throughout the world, sipping fragrant, steaming tea is a time-honored way to tap the healing properties of botanical remedies. Here are four recommended by MDs and natural health experts:

1 **VALERIAN PLUS LEMON BALM TEA FOR ANXIETY** Tea made from valerian root relaxes the nerves. Think of it as very weak Valium.

—**ROBERTA LEE**, MD, ASSISTANT CLINICAL PROFESSOR OF MEDICINE AT BANNER/ UNIVERSITY OF ARIZONA HEALTHCARE SYSTEM; CLINICAL FACULTY, PRIMARY CARE LINE AT THE SOUTHERN ARIZONA VETERANS ADMINISTRATION HEATHCARE SYSTEM IN TUCSON, ARIZONA; AND AUTHOR OF *THE SUPERSTRESS SOLUTION*

WHY IT WORKS Research suggests that combining valerian with lemon balm creates a mild natural sedative for some people. The lemon balm also tempers valerian's bitterness.

2 **PEPPERMINT TEA: TUMMY SOOTHER AND DECONGESTANT** Breathing the steam from a hot cuppa could open a stuffy nose. *(Ahh, I can breathe!)*

WHY IT WORKS Peppermint relaxes the muscles responsible for stomach cramps and may help with gas and diarrhea. The menthol in peppermint also acts as a decongestant, according to Peggy Kotsopoulos, registered holistic nutritionist and author of *Kitchen Cures: Revolutionize Your Health with Foods that Heal*

3 **LICORICE ROOT TEA: RELIEF FOR SORE THROATS** "Licorice root soothes mucous membranes in the throat," says Kotsopoulos. It also tastes pleasantly sweet. But to be on the safe side, skip licorice root tea if you're pregnant or breastfeeding, or have cardiology issues. In large quantities, this herb can raise blood pressure.

WHY IT WORKS Licorice root has anti-inflammatory properties that can help reduce swelling and irritation.

"LAUGHTER YOGA" TAMES TENSION

Melting stress is easy anywhere with what I call the "Ho-Ho-Ho" meditation. It's a favorite technique with my clients. One mother of two uses it when she goes shopping with her children. The tension of kids, stores, and crowds melts away if she does this while they stand in line.

It's simple. Close your eyes. Smile. Let go of your to-do list and worries, and focus your mind on the present. Now say this out loud: *Ha-ha! Ho-ho! Hee-hee!* Briefly picture a jolly Santa if you need to. You may feel silly, but you'll switch from irritation to giggles in a flash.

—SUSAN ALBERS, PSYD, CLINICAL PSYCHOLOGIST AT THE CLEVELAND CLINIC WOOSTER FAMILY HEALTH CENTER AND *NEW YORK TIMES* BEST-SELLING AUTHOR OF *EAT Q: UNLOCK THE WEIGHT-LOSS POWER OF EMOTIONAL INTELLIGENCE*

WHY IT WORKS →

"This technique is based on what's called laughter yoga, or Hasya yoga. Studies show that this fun practice helps boost your immune system and relieve stress. Making laughing noises gets the positive neurotransmitters in your brain flowing," says Albers. "The simple principle is that your body responds positively to your own laughter, even if you start it artificially. Upbeat feelings increase and bad moods fade away."

Laughter yoga doesn't just feel good. It has deeper benefits. At India's Bangalore University, people who participated in giggle sessions seven times in 18 days had significant drops in their blood pressure, heart rate, and levels of the stress hormone cortisol. And in a University of Wisconsin study, people who took a 15-minute laughter yoga class daily for two weeks became more optimistic, assertive, and motivated.

WHICH NATURAL FLU STOPPERS WORK?

In flu season, everyone wants to know if *Oscillococcinum*—a homeopathic therapy found in health food stores and many pharmacies—cures the flu. A small number of studies suggest that it may reduce how long the flu lasts, but only by a few hours. Not impressive.

But another popular flu remedy I get asked about is Sambucol, a brand of elderberry syrup. In one study, people who took it felt better an average of four days faster than those who took a placebo. There is not enough evidence to suggest that it can *prevent* colds or the flu. But feeling better that much faster is a good thing.

Bottom line is, while both *Oscillococcinum* and Sambucol may have immune-boosting properties, more research needs to be done.

If you decide to try either one, check with your doctor first. They're not recommended for babies or pregnant women, and can also interact with certain medications.

—MALLIKA MARSHALL, MD, URGENT CARE PHYSICIAN AT MASSACHUSETTS GENERAL HOSPITAL AND MEDICAL REPORTER AT CBS BOSTON'S WBZ-TV

 → Sambucol, or elderberry syrup, may have some antiviral properties that can ease symptoms," says Marshall. Also, she says, "I tell friends who want natural relief for flu symptoms that their best bets are saltwater gargles to soothe a sore throat and neti pot rinses to help with nasal congestion" (see page 99).

ANSWERS TO
ALTERNATIVE MEDICINE SMARTS

1 | **C.** While Tibetan monks and long-time practitioners may meditate for an hour or more, you can get benefits in just a few minutes—especially if you're new to meditation. Work up from five to even just 10 minutes a day and enjoy the stress-dissipating difference. *See page 84.*

2 | **A.** Elderberry syrup (sold as Sambucol, among other brands) has some antiviral properties. This may explain why, in one study, it helped people with flu feel better four days faster than a placebo did. Although it doesn't seem to prevent the flu, feeling better that much faster is a good thing. *See page 89.*

3 | **C.** Acupuncture has plenty of science behind it. This alternative healing modality can ease a wide variety of health conditions, and some top docs schedule appointments to "get needled" as a preventive health tune-up. *See page 81.*

4 | **B.** Pressing on the skin just below the arch of your eyebrows can ease headache pain, and it's hardly your body's only pressure point. Do-it-yourself acupressure works like acupuncture—without the needles—to stimulate areas that keep your body's energy flowing. This healing art can help lift your mood and ease neck pain, too. *See page 85.*

5 | **A.** Natural-healing experts suggest keeping a tube of calendula cream around to treat minor skin irritations and rashes . . . or having an easy-to-grow aloe plant on a windowsill. Gel from inside a broken-off piece of the plant helps small burns and inflammation heal. *See page 86.*

6 | **C.** It doesn't get any cheaper, easier, or faster than self-massage with a tennis ball. This works so well that one top researcher who studies massage and has demonstrated its pain-relieving benefits keeps a tennis ball handy for quick rub-downs. *See page 83.*

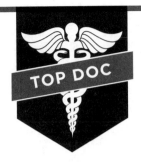

TOP DOC

REMEMBER THESE FIVE ALTERNATIVE MEDICINE SECRETS

Top docs' enthusiasm for alternative medicine is surprisingly strong—and we bet it's motivated you to explore its many healing options. With so many possibilities to choose from, let these guidelines help you decide which ones to try:

1 **START WITH SIMPLE, AT-HOME TECHNIQUES.** Not ready to get needled by an acupuncturist? Try do-it-yourself acupressure. Can't swing an hour-long massage? Explore self-massage, starting with just an ordinary tennis ball. Not only can remedies like these work surprisingly well but also they're instantly available. No need to find a practitioner or wait for an appointment!

2 **INTERESTED IN HERBAL MEDICINE? CHOOSE GENTLE BOTANICALS.** Calendula cream for irritated skin. Elderberry syrup for a case of the flu. Sticking with gentle remedies like these—and the others recommended in this chapter—can help you get results without raising your risk for adverse reactions. Be wary of high-potency herbal products, and avoid taking remedies for long periods of time, unless recommended by a trained natural healer who is personally treating you.

3 **TELL YOUR DOCTOR WHAT YOU'RE DOING.** She or he can help you assess whether a remedy is working for you and alert you if it might interfere with other treatments. While physicians can do this for themselves, the rest of us need a little help.

4 **PRACTICE MEDITATIVE BREATHING FOR JUST FIVE MINUTES TODAY.** Repeat tomorrow. It eases stress, improves your mood, and has a slew of other proven health benefits. If you explore just one new "alternative" therapy, consider this the one.

5 **LAUGH.** Really. It's the ultimate fun, do-anywhere "add-on" therapy for a brighter mood, lower blood pressure, stronger immunity, and instant anxiety relief.

BEAT COLDS & FLU

IF YOU WANT TO AVOID GETTING COLDS OR FLU—or, for that matter, much of anything else—top docs recommend a variety of methods. For starters, flu shots, which slash the risk of a nasty case of influenza at least in half—goodbye chills, fever, coughing, and just plain feeling awful. Top docs recommend getting vaccinated against the flu yearly. Just 41% of American adults and 56% of kids get vaccinated, even though it's recommended for almost everyone over six months old. What makes docs so motivated to tell patients to get their flu shots? They know the score.

- ▶ **SHEER NUMBERS.** The vaccine prevents an estimated 6.6 million cases of the flu every year, and they intend to be among them.
- ▶ **PNEUMONIA.** It also cuts the risk for serious flu complications, like pneumonia. This keeps an estimated 79,000 people out of the hospital each year, including docs.
- ▶ **DYING.** It shrinks the risk of succumbing to the flu by up to 28%.
- ▶ **HEART ATTACKS AND STROKE.** Finally, more and more evidence shows that the flu shot cuts the odds for having a wintertime heart attack or stroke by 50%—most likely by reducing flu-related stress and inflammation on your heart and arteries.

Top docs are determined to help their patients avoid rotten colds, too. In one survey, 86% of hospital physicians washed up as recommended, scrubbing for at least 15 seconds before and after attending to patients. Many tell their patients to use similar techniques—surprisingly, 70% of us don't lather up even after using the restroom (!), a primo place for nasty viruses and bacteria. At best, many Americans just rinse.

As a result, many of us can expect to sneeze through 62 million colds per year and face up to a one in five chance for catching the flu. Don't be one of them. Ahead are top docs' tips for staying well while everyone around you is keeling over—and how you can get fast relief on the occasions when you're under the weather.

TEST YOUR
COLD AND FLU DEFENSES

You don't have time to be sick. That's why top docs believe you should be diligent about fending off cold and flu viruses. They know which remedies you should grab—fast—when symptoms kick up, and they never stop spreading the word about the importance of getting a flu shot. Are you up on the latest ways to prevent nasty upper respiratory tract infections and keep them in check?

1 **True or False:** Blowing your nose the wrong way can make a cold worse.

2 **Pregnant women should get a flu shot because:**

a. Moms-to-be are at higher risk for flu-related complications.

b. It protects their babies for about six months after they're born.

c. Both.

d. Neither. Women should not get flu shots if they're pregnant.

3 **Your risk of catching a cold on an airplane is this much higher than it is on the ground:**

a. Twice as high

b. 10 times higher

c. 23 times higher

4 **True or false:** Though it's rare, you can catch the flu from the flu vaccine.

5 **This common kitchen ingredient can cut your risk for catching a cold or the flu—and for developing a secondary sinus infection if you do get one:**

a. Cayenne pepper

b. Table salt

c. Sage

6 **If you've had the flu and your fever has broken, how long should you wait before going out into the world again?**

a. 24 hours

b. 48 hours

c. There's no need to wait. You're no longer contagious.

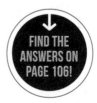

FIND THE ANSWERS ON PAGE 106!

FIGHT, FIGHT, FIGHT A COLD

Whenever friends tell me they feel like they're coming down with an upper respiratory infection and are going to the doctor for antibiotics, I urge them to reconsider. Antibiotics don't work if you have a virus, and most upper respiratory infections are viral. If someone's really ill, that's different. Their physician can decide whether antibiotics are needed.

But otherwise, I tell them to do what I do when I feel something coming on: Mix together equal parts olive oil and raw honey, then add generous amounts of black pepper, cinnamon, ginger, and turmeric. There's no exact recipe, just season to taste.

I dose myself with one teaspoon a day to ease a sore throat and shorten sick time. It tastes great, makes my throat feel better, and helps reduce down time.

—LESLIE MENDOZA TEMPLE, MD, MEDICAL DIRECTOR OF THE INTEGRATIVE MEDICINE PROGRAM AT NORTHSHORE UNIVERSITY HEALTHSYSTEM, NEW YORK

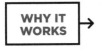 **WHY IT WORKS** → "Raw honey has antiviral and antibacterial properties," says Mendoza Temple, "and some research shows that turmeric, an anti-inflammatory, can help prevent or relieve a cold."

THAT'S NOT ALL:

▶ **BLACK PEPPER** does more than lend a spicy zing to this remedy; there's evidence that it spurs your immune system's germ-destroying natural killer cells to work harder.

▶ **CINNAMON** isn't just a flavor star; it also has unusually high levels of plant compounds called polyphenols, which rev up your body's antioxidant defenses, reports the Department of Agriculture.

▶ **GINGER** extracts inhibit the growth of staph and strep bacteria, and a recent study found that fresh ginger slows the growth of human respiratory syncytial virus, a common virus that causes symptoms that mimic the common cold.

SET UP A SICKROOM

I sleep in another room when I am ill. When someone in the household has the flu—or anything else contagious—we try to keep away from each other. This is one of the ways to stop transmission of the infection.

It's okay for one or two people to act as caregivers to the sick one. Just touch as few things as possible when you're in the sickroom, including the patient, and don't volunteer for caregiving duty if you're pregnant or already have a medical condition. Always make sure to wash your hands after exiting the room or set up an anti-microbial hand sanitizer just outside the room. Catching the flu is bad enough, but spreading it puts others at risk for illness, missed work or school, and potential complications.

Finally, everyone should wash their hands constantly!

—WILBUR H. CHEN, MD, MS, FACP, ASSOCIATE PROFESSOR OF MEDICINE AT THE UNIVERSITY OF MARYLAND SCHOOL OF MEDICINE AND DIRECTOR OF THE UNIVERSITY'S TRAVELERS' HEALTH CLINIC

SET UP A SICKROOM WITH THESE ITEMS, RECOMMENDED BY THE CENTERS FOR DISEASE CONTROL AND PREVENTION:

✔ An alcohol-based hand rub

✔ Plenty of tissues

✔ A trash can lined with a plastic bag for easy, no-touch disposal

✔ Plenty of liquids—keep drinks in a cooler or pitcher; designate cups for hot liquids for the sick family member

✔ A humidifier

✔ Face masks—the sick person should wear one any time he or she leaves the room (say, to use the bathroom). If there's more than one bathroom, designate one as a flu zone and have everyone else use the other.

WHY IT WORKS → Germs can live on doorknobs and other hard surfaces for up to 48 hours, which is reason enough to steer clear of sick people—but you're much more likely to get infected from airborne germs. A direct hit from a cough or sneeze is usually far more potent than droplets that have been sitting around on a doorknob (phone, mouse) for even a few minutes. Keep your distance from sneezing, coughing adults and kids, recommends Jon Abramson, MD, professor of pediatrics at Wake Forest School of Medicine and medical advisor for the nonprofit Families Fighting Flu.

WASH, WASH, WASH

Frequent hand washing is always important, but especially in cold-and-flu season and especially when you're in public places or around sick people.

Use alcohol-based hand sanitizers in a pinch, but when good old-fashioned soap and water is available, it's the best. Make sure to wash around and under your fingernails and rings, as well as between your fingers. These areas are frequently missed, and that's where germs tend to hide out.

—GINA M. SOLOMON, MD, CLINICAL PROFESSOR OF MEDICINE AT THE UNIVERSITY OF CALIFORNIA, SAN FRANCISCO

Frequent hand washing is still the best cold prevention ever simply because it gets rid of germs before they can get inside your body. Yet just 5% of people wash their hands well enough to kill infection-causing germs, found a Michigan State University study of 3,749 people in public restrooms.

Work up a soapy lather and rub for 20 seconds, the time it takes to sing the "Happy Birthday" song twice. Don't forget those often-neglected spots that Solomon targets. Rinse well and dry with a clean towel or under a hand dryer. You're good to go.

PREGNANT?
GET A FLU SHOT *NOW*

As the dad of a new baby myself, I can't tell you how upset I was recently when I was working in an ICU and had to treat a critically ill mom-to-be who later died of flu complications. Now I say this to every pregnant woman I know: If you get influenza, you are at a higher risk of complications and death. And even if you come through okay, your illness could hurt your baby-to-be, especially if you get the flu during your third trimester.

Doctors still don't fully understand why the flu is so dangerous to pregnant women and their babies, but it most likely involves your inability to breathe properly. You can't possibly pass enough oxygen to your unborn child if you're struggling for breath yourself. That can harm the fetus in many different ways.

So if you're pregnant, absolutely get a flu shot. And if you start feeling flu-ish, call your doctor and discuss treatment options, just to be safe.

—CAMERON WOLFE, MD, INFECTIOUS DISEASE SPECIALIST AT DUKE UNIVERSITY MEDICAL CENTER IN DURHAM, NORTH CAROLINA

WHY IT WORKS → A flu shot in pregnancy protects babies from birth until they're about six months old, says the CDC. That window of protection is important, because babies younger than six months cannot have the shot themselves. If you have your baby before getting a flu shot, get one anyway. It's safe for breastfeeding moms and nursing babies, and protecting yourself lowers your newborn's risk. Everyone in your household or who cares for your baby should also be vaccinated.

KEEP COLDS FROM BECOMING SINUS INFECTIONS

If you have a cold, congestion is a major issue. What I preach to everyone is "Keep your nose open!" If you can breathe through your nose, it reduces the likelihood of sinus infections and other secondary complications. When I have a dry mouth and realize I'm not breathing through my nose because one or both sides are blocked, I reach for a decongestant spray right away.

For most people, it's okay to use a decongestant nasal spray as directed for three to five days and it will bring tremendous relief without causing rebound congestion.

—GAILEN D. MARSHALL JR., MD, PHD, PROFESSOR OF MEDICINE AND DIRECTOR OF THE DIVISION OF CLINICAL IMMUNOLOGY AND ALLERGY AT THE UNIVERSITY OF MISSISSIPPI MEDICAL CENTER, JACKSON

Just don't rely on a decongestant for longer than recommended. Prolonged use can backfire, causing structures inside your nose to swell hours later— that's what "rebound congestion" is. This can lead to overuse and dependence.

If you're still congested after three to five days, stop using the decongestant spray. Switch to a saline nose rinse or try guaifenesin, an over-the-counter mucus thinner that works for some people. Dislike nasal sprays? Use decongestant pills instead.

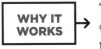 "Don't wait," says Marshall. "The sooner you use a decongestant, the better. It prevents your nasal turbinates— three pairs of long, thin bones covered with a thin layer of tissue inside the walls of your nose—from swelling and blocking the openings to your sinuses. That's key, because the viruses and bacteria that cause sinus infections thrive when mucus gets trapped by congestion."

SMOKERS: LET THE FLU HELP YOU QUIT

Few smokers realize that smoking is particularly dangerous if they get the flu. Cigarettes do a number on your immune system anyway, but they also negate essential mechanisms that help your lungs fight a virus. Specifically, smoking disables little hairs on the lungs' surface that act like a broom to sweep away infection.

The result can be a life-threatening complication such as viral pneumonia or, worse, a bacterial super-virus that's dangerously resistant to antibiotics. That scary danger should make anyone kick the habit.

—ARNOLD MONTO, MD, PROFESSOR OF EPIDEMIOLOGY AT THE UNIVERSITY OF MICHIGAN SCHOOL OF PUBLIC HEALTH, ANN ARBOR

 Feeling too sick to smoke when you have the flu is actually an advantage. By the time you start to feel better, you've already gotten through the first few days of withdrawal. Instead of reaching for a cigarette, reach for a nicotine patch and call your doctor for more help. The most effective quitting strategy includes taking an antidepressant such as bupropion early on because it eases nicotine cravings; continue using nicotine patches, too, and get support from a counselor or support group.

The rewards of quitting pile up fast. Within 12 hours, levels of carbon monoxide in your bloodstream fall to normal. Within 14 days, your lung function begins to improve. Within one year, your extra risk for heart disease is cut in half. And within five years, the threat of cancers of your mouth, throat, esophagus, and bladder drops 50%.

THREE WAYS TO BOOST YOUR COLD AND FLU IQ

Heed this important stay-well advice from two top infectious-disease docs.

1 **GET ENOUGH SLEEP.** It's one of the best but least-known ways to stay well. It can really help keep you cold-proof and flu-free. Getting enough sleep helps make your immune system more active and puts it into "ready to fight" mode.

WHY IT WORKS Too little sleep triggers a falloff of up to 30% in the activity of your immune system's natural killer cells, reports a Stockholm study. People who regularly get less than seven hours of shut-eye a night are nearly three times more likely to catch a cold than those who get eight or more hours, according to research from Carnegie Mellon University, according to Stacey Rizza, MD, infectious-disease specialist at the Mayo Clinic in Rochester, Minnesota.

2 **GET FLU SHOTS ASAP.** Why? Simple math: You're protected for the whole six-month flu season—October through March—not just part of it. Also, it can take up to two weeks for your body to develop protective antibodies to the virus, so the earlier, the better.

WHY IT HELPS While the vaccine isn't 100% effective, it reduces your chances of getting sick by 50 to 90%, depending on how closely that year's vaccine and virus match up. If you catch the flu anyway, it most likely won't be as bad, says Jon Abramson, MD, professor of pediatrics at Wake Forest School of Medicine and medical advisor for the nonprofit Families Fighting Flu.

3 **KNOW THE DIFFERENCE BETWEEN A HORRIBLE COLD AND THE FLU.** Usually fever is the best indication. If an adult has severe cold-like symptoms plus a fever of 101°F or higher, it's a good bet it's the flu, says Abramson. Other telltale signs include body aches, chills, and feeling too wiped out to drag yourself out of bed.

WHY IT MATTERS Don't assume a fever means it's a case of the flu in kids. Many things can cause fevers in young children and merit a call to the doctor.

10-SECOND SOLUTIONS

THINK ZINC

Does zinc really help shorten a cold? Yes, if you act fast. Multiple studies show that zinc can minimize symptoms and often shorten a cold's life span. Zinc helps stop the virus from reproducing and revs up your immune cells as well. The minute you start sniffling or notice a scratchy throat, start sucking on zinc lozenges. Then follow every-few-hours dosage directions for up to five days.

—**STACEY RIZZA**, MD, INFECTIOUS DISEASE SPECIALIST AT THE MAYO CLINIC IN ROCHESTER, MINNESOTA

FIGHT FLU FAST

If you suspect the flu, call your doc pronto. She or he can prescribe antiviral medications that can cut your miserable sick time in half, especially if you act fast and take them within two days of your symptoms starting.

STAY HOME!

You can spread the flu for up to a day before you develop symptoms and even if you don't have the typically severe flu symptoms. Just mild body aches or a cough could mean you have the virus—and you could give a full-blown case to someone else with a weaker immune system. So be nice: Avoid physical contact with others until you're sure you're okay. If you eventually get sick, stay home from work until your symptoms really start to fade and at least 24 hours after any fever breaks. It's good for you and your colleagues!

—**REKHA MURTHY**, MD, VICE PRESIDENT FOR MEDICAL AFFAIRS AND ASSOCIATE CHIEF MEDICAL OFFICER AT CEDARS-SINAI IN LOS ANGELES

DON'T FEAR FLU SHOTS

One of the most common questions I'm asked by my friends is whether you can get the flu from the vaccine. I always answer, "No!" But even my husband is convinced that the head cold he swears he often gets after the flu vaccine was caused by the shot. My own husband! The truth is that the flu shot contains inactive virus that *cannot* cause the flu.

—**MALLIKA MARSHALL**, MD, URGENT CARE PHYSICIAN AT MASSACHUSETTS GENERAL HOSPITAL AND MEDICAL REPORTER AT CBS BOSTON'S WBZ-TV

ABOUT TO SNEEZE?

Cover your nose and mouth with a tissue when you cough or sneeze, then throw the tissue away *immediately*, urges the CDC. No time to grab a tissue? Cover your face with the crook of your elbow, Dracula-style.

THINK BEYOND THE ORANGE

"There are many other fruits and veggies to get your vitamin C from! Strawberries, kiwis, broccoli, cauliflower, tomatoes, Brussels sprouts, melon . . . these are just a few of the vitamin C–packed foods you can eat that are chock-full of the nutrient. That said—unless you're *deficient* in vitamin C (almost none of us are!) eating more of them won't help you . . . but since they're all hydrating and fiber-rich, incorporating a little extra can help you fill up on deliciously soothing foods."

—**JACLYN LONDON**, MS, RD, GOOD HOUSEKEEPING NUTRITION DIRECTOR

NOSE BLOWING 101

Less than half of the people we see in the clinic know how to blow their nose properly. So we teach them how, because we've found it lowers their risk for developing a secondary sinus infection after a cold.

The right way: Close one nostril by pushing on the side of your nose and *gently* blowing out on the other side for a few seconds. Then switch sides. You may have to repeat the process, but it really helps you get everything out.

—GAILEN D. MARSHALL JR, MD, PHD, PROFESSOR OF MEDICINE AND DIRECTOR OF THE DIVISION OF CLINICAL IMMUNOLOGY AND ALLERGY AT THE UNIVERSITY OF MISSISSIPPI MEDICAL CENTER, JACKSON

WHY IT WORKS → "When you blow your nose hard, you get what docs call a reflex nasal obstruction," Marshall explains. "Think about the last time you had a big sneeze. For a few seconds or even minutes afterward your nose probably felt like it got stopped up, but then it opened up again. That's reflex nasal obstruction. Its purpose is to keep you from *not* breathing back in what you've made such an effort to expel. But when you blow hard frequently you can actually make congestion worse, and that sets you up for an infection."

Forceful nose blowing can also up your risk of a sinus infection a second way. A study at the University of Virginia found that honking and hard nose blowing creates a vacuum that propels icky snot backward into your sinuses. A single, strong honk could send nearly a quarter teaspoon of mucus in the wrong direction. Yuck.

HOW NOT TO GET SICK WHEN YOU FLY

All that airport angst about catching colds on planes? It's not travelers' nerves. You're 23 times (!) more likely to pick up a cold in the air than on the ground, found an analysis of more than 1,100 airline passengers. But guess what? It's not the recirculated air in the plane that's to blame. Passengers are just as likely to experience cold symptoms if the cabin contains fresh air, according to a study at the University of California, San Francisco.

The culprit is probably the low humidity in aircraft cabins, for two reasons: First, it dries out the sticky mucus in your nose, compromising its ability to trap and eliminate viruses. Second, most cold-causing viruses survive better when humidity is low, which increases the chance of a virus spreading from passenger to passenger.

—MARTIN B. HOCKING, PHD, CO-AUTHOR OF THE COLD STUDY AND PROFESSOR EMERITUS OF ENVIRONMENTAL CHEMISTRY AT THE UNIVERSITY OF VICTORIA, BRITISH COLUMBIA

How to fight an in-flight cold? Try saline nasal drops, sprays, gels, or moisturizing nasal swabs to keep nasal passages from drying up. And stay hydrated.

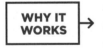

WHY IT WORKS → Anything that combats drying nasal passages—especially during flights lasting more than two hours, Hocking says—not only helps you breathe more comfortably but also prevents the congestion and dry nasal crusting that viruses love.

ANSWERS TO
COLD AND FLU DEFENSES

1 | **TRUE.** Your mom was right about this one. Forceful nose blowing is counterproductive. It can force germy gunk deeper into your sinuses, promoting infection. Better blowing technique: Gently, one nostril at a time. *See page 104.*

2 | **C.** If you're pregnant, might be, or are just trying, be sure to get a flu shot. It's proven to shield you *and* your baby from potentially life-threatening complications of the flu. *See page 98.*

3 | **C.** It's not urban lore. You're way more likely to catch the sniffles on a plane. The reason: Low in-flight humidity, which dries out the mucous membranes in your nose and sinuses so they can't immobilize germs. Your best defense: saline nose sprays throughout that plane trip. *See page 105.*

4 | **FALSE.** The virus in the vaccine is inactive and cannot give you influenza. If you do come down with flu soon after getting your shot, you were most likely exposed to the flu virus before you got the vaccine or soon after. It takes a couple of weeks to build immunity. *See page 103.*

5 | **B.** Dissolving a little table salt in warm water for gargling or to use as a nose rinse can cut your risk of an upper respiratory tract infection by 60% and reduce the odds that your cold will morph into a sinus infection by a whopping 72%. *See page 107.*

6 | **A.** Once your fever cools, you may feel ready to get back to normal life. But the world isn't ready for you. You could still pass the virus along to others, so hang out at home for another day just to be on the safe side. *See page 102.*

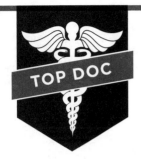

REMEMBER THESE FIVE COLD AND FLU SECRETS

Fight colds and flu like a top doc with these five at-a-glance strategies for preventing and treating those miserable upper respiratory infections:

1 **WASH YOUR HANDS THE RIGHT WAY.** Lather up with soap and warm water, scrub for 20 seconds—especially around rings and fingernails—rinse well and dry. It may be the most effective do-it-yourself protection against cold and flu viruses.

2 **PROTECT YOURSELF AND YOU'LL PROTECT THE PEOPLE YOU LOVE.** We can't say it enough: Get a flu shot. The more people who do, the better. By getting your whole family vaccinated, you're also protecting your kids' friends and teachers, your own friends and colleagues, and your kids' elderly grandparents.

3 **KEEP THIS ARSENAL ON HAND.** Table salt, for mixing up mild salt water for an infection-fighting gargle or nasal rinse. Zinc lozenges to cut short cold symptoms. Honey, olive oil, black pepper, and ginger for an immune-revving tonic.

4 **QUARANTINE THE SICK PERSON, EVEN IF IT'S YOU.** Setting up a sickroom—and staying home in it even if you really want to go back to work when symptoms first fade—can keep your family and co-workers from catching the flu from you.

5 **COVER COUGHS AND SNEEZES, BUT NOT WITH YOUR HAND.** Droplets propelled through the air by a forceful *achoo!* are more potent than germs hanging out on doorknobs. Sneeze into a tissue or the crook of your elbow—and retreat fast when others are doing the sneezing.

NO-FRILLS
FITNESS

AT BEST, ABOUT 35% OF AMERICANS FIT IN SOME VIGOROUS PHYSICAL ACTIVITY during the week. About 18% of us fit in the recommended levels of weekly fitness (150 minutes of moderate activity or 75 minutes of vigorous activity plus two strength-training sessions weekly), according to a recent National Health Information poll. But top docs recommend hard-charging exercise—the kind that raises your heart rate and burns fat, thereby controlling weight and increasing cardiovascular fitness. And they're more likely to use whatever time is available—any place, any time of day—to fit exercise in. Go for a run at 5:30 a.m.? Park far off and speed-walk daily from car to office? Keep fitness gear at work and *use* it? Top docs do all that and more, as you'll see.

They enjoy it, too. In a 2014 survey of American physicians, 70% rated exercise their second most favorite leisure activity. Spending time with family was number one, but fitness was ahead of travel, reading, going to movies and concerts, and enjoying food and wine.

Docs don't go in for trendy fitness classes at fancy gyms, either. What do they like to do best? Here's what healers told Medscape in a 2012 survey:

- ▶ **71% walk**
- ▶ **28% rate weight lifting and strength training as tops**
- ▶ **29% of female docs and about 9% of male docs are fans of yoga, Pilates, tai chi, or martial arts**
- ▶ **24% of male docs and about 8% of female docs like tennis, golf, and/or other sports**
- ▶ **20% of females and about 4% of males dance for exercise**
- ▶ **16% love winter sports, like skiing and skating**
- ▶ **10% rank water sports (canoeing, kayaking, sailing) as their top activity.**

Finally, what keeps them motivated? Physicians probably know better than anyone that working out helps prevent disease, stay slim, and keep brain power high. So while docs don't have any more time than you do, they make it happen anyway—getting up earlier, using buddy systems, turning fitness into a family affair, stowing exercise stuff in cars for spur-of-the-moment workouts, streaming fitness workouts when traveling, and more.

Here are the ways they do it that will work for you, too.

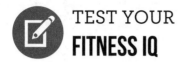

TEST YOUR
FITNESS IQ

Sometimes, all it takes to make a new exercise routine stick is having the right music in your smartphone . . . or keeping a few inexpensive, muscle-building resistance bands handy . . . or knowing one *really* short routine there's always time to do. Simple enablers like these make all the difference. Take this quiz about the little secrets that add up to big exercise success, then read on to learn more.

1 Exercising early helps you stick with it, but how much? In one survey, what percentage of morning exercisers were still working out a year later?

a. 28%

b. 53%

c. 75%

2 Want to blast midlife belly fat? Do this:

a. Walk for 60 minutes every day.

b. Take up power yoga.

c. Exercise for 22 minutes a day—walk four or five times a week; do strength training two or three times a week.

3 The best way to build muscle is to:

a. Use weight machines at the gym every Tuesday, Thursday, and Saturday.

b. Use resistance bands or hand weights at home about three times a week.

c. Do one of these every day.

4 If you're sick, follow this fitness rule:

a. No workouts for 72 hours after a fever returns to normal.

b. If you can lace up your sneakers, it's okay to exercise.

c. Get back to your routine a week after you start feeling better.

5 To get kids to spend exercise time with you:

a. Go on long fitness walks, runs, or bike rides together.

b. Sign them up for tennis, golf, volleyball, or weight-lifting lessons.

c. Do stop-and-go activities together—shell-hunting beach walks, backyard ball games, critter-spotting nature trails.

6 Use music to increase your exercise motivation by picking tunes that:

a. You love and build from slow to fast

b. Have a tempo that matches your heart rate

c. Are high-energy from the beginning

FIND THE ANSWERS ON PAGE 126!

WORK OUT EARLY

I'm a big advocate of exercise, and I totally practice what I preach to my patients—although I always say to them, "You don't have to do as much as I do or as early as I do it!" I get up at 5 a.m. every day and swim a mile, run three miles, or bike 12 miles. I also lift weights 5 days a week. To do this, I go to bed at 9 p.m. and am usually asleep by 9:15.

To maintain good health for the long term, ideally you'd aim for an hour of physical activity every day. If you walk at a 20-minute mile pace, that's a three-mile walk. But if you have absolutely no time some days, just do 10 minutes. Everyone can find 10 minutes.

My biggest message is, try to do it in the morning. Morning exercise makes you physically and mentally alert, so you're more likely to be at peak creativity and productivity for the rest of the day.

—ARTHUR J. MOLLEN, DO, OSTEOPATHIC FAMILY PHYSICIAN IN SCOTTSDALE, ARIZONA, AND AUTHOR OF SEVERAL BOOKS, INCLUDING *HEALTHONOMICS: THE HANDBOOK FOR BALANCING YOUR PHYSICAL AND FINANCIAL CHECKBOOKS*

Long-standing research also suggests that being active in the morning, rather than later in the day, promotes better sleep at night. However, new evidence shows that afternoon workouts may do a better job of *lengthening* your sleep time. The overall consensus, though, is to just do it, no matter when you squeeze it in.

WHY IT WORKS "A study I did with my patients supported research others have done: 75% of morning exercisers stick with it for at least a year, compared to 50% who exercise at lunch and 25% who work out at the end of the day," Mollen says. "Getting in your workout first thing, before there are other demands on your time, makes it easier to get it done regularly."

SHIMMY-SHIMMY, SHAKE-SHAKE-SHAKE!

I recently took a Zumba class for the first time and was surprised by how sexy I felt afterward! Physiologically, I realized it was the result of moving my hips and back so much, plus keeping that blood flowing can decrease vaginal dryness. I also knew that doing this class consistently would give me flexibility and strength, which is important as you age. So I resolved to attend Zumba classes three times a week—and I've stuck with it. When I can't make the class or I'm traveling, I work out with Zumba DVDs.

And talk about benefits for a relationship. If my husband had been around after that first class, I would have jumped him!

—HILDA Y. HUTCHERSON, MD, PROFESSOR OF OBSTETRICS AND GYNECOLOGY AT COLUMBIA UNIVERSITY MEDICAL CENTER AND AUTHOR OF *WHAT YOUR MOTHER NEVER TOLD YOU ABOUT SEX AND PLEASURE*

WHY IT WORKS → In Spanish, the word *Zumba* means "buzz like a bee, and move fast." This catchy, calorie-burning, wildly popular exer-dance has caught on with an estimated 12 million people worldwide. The moves and the music—a mash-up of salsa, merengue, reggaeton, and flamenco—feel more like a party than a workout, but a study found that Zumba is serious exercise. In sessions that last about 30 to 50 minutes, dancers burn an average of 370 calories per session and their heart rate hits 80% of maximum. That's right in the recommended zone for increasing cardiovascular fitness, say researchers at the University of Wisconsin–La Crosse.

BEAT EXERCISE BOREDOM

I struggle with consistent exercise, even though I see the effects of slacking off in my patients and myself. So I do what I tell them to do: schedule it into the workday. I *plan* a brisk walk during lunch. Or I replace every coffee break with a fitness break—I've actually put a mini trampoline in my office to do this. It also lets me get moving when the mood strikes.

But what motivates me most is watching movies at home. I only let myself do that when I'm pedaling the elliptical. I'll get back on the machine just to finish a movie!

—HILARY TINDLE, MD, ASSISTANT PROFESSOR OF MEDICINE, DIVISION OF GENERAL INTERNAL MEDICINE, AT THE UNIVERSITY OF PITTSBURGH SCHOOL OF MEDICINE

> **WHY IT WORKS** → Commitment may be the key to a successful fitness regimen, but sticking with the same routine over and over is not. In fact, if you do the same workout day in and day out, your body begins to master it, your calories burned begin to dwindle, your progress starts to stall, and your commitment wimps out. Use Tindle's solution: Switch things up!

THREE EASY WAYS TO DO THAT:

▶ **VARY YOUR PACE.** Instead of walking at the same steady speed, do interval training. Alternate 30- to 60-second bursts of very fast walking or jogging with doing several minutes at your regular pace. You'll burn more fat and calories, and get fitter.

▶ **CROSS-TRAIN.** If you *always* bike, swim, weight train, or do yoga, why not try other types of exercise? You'll work different muscles, burn plenty of calories, and get the same great sense of well-being afterward.

▶ **COMPETE.** Okay, you're not headed for the Olympics. Neither are we. But how about signing up for a local 5K hike or bike ride? It provides a goal to work toward and a fun "I did it!" celebration at the finish line.

BUILD SLEEK, SEXY MUSCLE

I love elastic exercise bands. They're a great way to get strong without weights or machines, especially when you're traveling or stuck at your desk all day. I try to do eight to 10 different exercises two or three times a week, hitting all the major muscle groups. There are good workouts all over the Web—check the American Council on Exercise site at www.acefitness.org.

—MARILYN MOFFAT, PT, DPT, PHD, PROFESSOR OF PHYSICAL THERAPY AT NEW YORK UNIVERSITY AND AUTHOR OF *AGE-DEFYING FITNESS: MAKING THE MOST OF YOUR BODY FOR THE REST OF YOUR LIFE*

"You can do the same exercises with elastic bands as you would with weights or machines and get a great workout and *great* results," says Moffat. Exercise bands come in different colors that represent resistance level. To find the right strengthener for you, select one at the store and do an exercise twice. Ask yourself if the effort is fairly light, somewhat hard, or hard. "Somewhat hard" is what you want. When you're working out, eight to 12 repetitions of each move should make the muscles you're using tired.

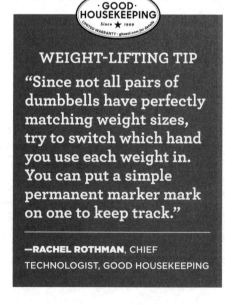

WEIGHT-LIFTING TIP

"Since not all pairs of dumbbells have perfectly matching weight sizes, try to switch which hand you use each weight in. You can put a simple permanent marker mark on one to keep track."

—RACHEL ROTHMAN, CHIEF TECHNOLOGIST, GOOD HOUSEKEEPING

STAY IN SHAPE ON THE ROAD

When I get to an airport, instead of plunking down at the gate I keep moving. By the time I get onto the plane, I've gotten in 30 minutes of fast walking. That can easily burn off a couple hundred calories.

—**TRAVIS STORK**, MD, EMERGENCY MEDICINE PHYSICIAN AND HOST OF THE EMMY AWARD–WINNING DAYTIME SHOW *THE DOCTORS*

Whether it's a business or pleasure trip, once you've reached your destination take the same approach there as Stork does to airports:

▶ **EXPLORE THE AREA WITH SNEAKERS ON.** Check with historical societies, architecture groups, and nature preserves about walking tours and hikes. Or take a guided running tour—you'll find them for many US cities at www. CityRunningTours.com.

▶ **CHECK OUT THE HOTEL FITNESS CENTER.** If there isn't one or it leaves something to be desired, find local gyms and print out a pass at www.GymTicket.com. If you belong to a fitness chain or the Y, ask about reciprocal guest privileges—you may be able to fit in a workout for just a few dollars.

▶ **OPEN YOUR LAPTOP.** Then type "free workout videos" into your browser. You'll find hundreds of convenient, no-cost routines. Looking for a 10-minute walking workout, 20 minutes of strength training, or a 30-minute yoga session? Type what you want to narrow the search and have at it! Always check with your doctor first and make sure workouts are from a trusted source.

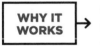 → Just doing a little can do a lot when you're on the road and juggling activities. You won't gain fitness, but you can maintain a nice level with even short bursts of activity— how about a brisk 10-minute walk before breakfast, then 10 minutes of easy strength-training moves in your room in the evening? You can do that! And it's enough to keep your metabolism humming, get your muscles moving, and let you arrive home guilt-free and ready to return to your regular routine.

MAKE-AHEAD LUNCHES CREATE TIME FOR EXERCISE

Food you prepare yourself is almost always healthier than food you buy. I always make lunch for me and my family. I invested in great insulated lunch bags, and spend 15 minutes the night before packing up tasty food in airtight containers. It might be leftover roast vegetables topped with crumbled feta, or a turkey sandwich with lettuce and tomato on whole-wheat bread. There is always a piece of fruit, and sometimes a homemade treat like an oatmeal cookie with chopped dates. This is a winner plan in every way: You have delicious food, you're not tempted by a vending machine, and the extra time saved by having lunch ready in the office can be spent stretching or going for a brisk walk.

—CAROLYN BERNSTEIN MD, FAHS, ASSISTANT PROFESSOR OF NEUROLOGY AT THE HARVARD-AFFILIATED BRIGHAM AND WOMEN'S HOSPITAL IN BOSTON AND AUTHOR OF *THE MIGRAINE BRAIN*

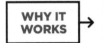 Having a ready-to-eat lunch on hand could give you an extra 15 to 30 minutes a day for exercising during your lunch break—time you might otherwise spend waiting in the cafeteria line at work or hopping in the car to go pick up a sandwich. A growing stack of research shows that even short periods of exercise can help you stay healthier and live longer.

TREAT YOUR HOME AS A GYM

If the weather's lousy, there are two easy ways of fitting in aerobic conditioning. Climbing stairs is one, but if you don't have stairs—or you're a fitness beginner—simply march in place. Bring your knees up to a point midway between the top of your hip bone and your normal knee level when standing. March as quickly as you can. Start with 10 to 15 seconds and build up to two minutes or more.

If you're reasonably fit and do have a flight of stairs, go for it! Start by doing two flights each up and down. Progress as your conditioning increases.

—MARILYN MOFFAT, PT, DPT, PHD, PROFESSOR OF PHYSICAL THERAPY AT NEW YORK UNIVERSITY AND AUTHOR OF *AGE-DEFYING FITNESS: MAKING THE MOST OF YOUR BODY FOR THE REST OF YOUR LIFE*

WHY IT WORKS → "Once you've built up some stair fitness, doing multiple flights is a terrific form of interval training," Moffat says. "I live on the 12th floor of an apartment building, and when it's pouring rain, I go up and down the internal stairway in my building, doing 10 flights six times. It's a *great* workout."

Women who climbed the stairs in their apartment buildings daily during an eight-week study saw their heart and lungs get 17% healthier *and* their heart-threatening bad LDL cholesterol drop 7%. What's more, climbing stairs (versus using a stair machine) and marching in place are high-impact activities that stimulate healthy bone growth and lower your fracture risk.

WORK OUT WHILE YOU WORK

I've worked at a treadmill desk for years to help me fit in 10,000 steps a day. I've discovered I can write at 1.7 miles per hour, type at 1.8 miles per hour, and read at 1.9 miles per hour! During conference calls, I get up to 3.3 miles per hour.

But you don't need a high-tech fitness desk, though they're great. There's plenty you can do to break up sitting time during the workday. The easiest strategy is just to get up every half hour and move for a few minutes—march in place while you're on the phone, walk to the water fountain, use the restroom farthest from your desk, or go talk to a coworker in person instead of sending an email.

 YOU CAN ALSO TRY THESE INEXPENSIVE FITNESS GIZMOS THAT ENGAGE YOUR MUSCLES AND BURN CALORIES:

✔ Sit on a large exercise ball instead of your desk chair for part of the day—the constant little balancing motions strengthen your core.

✔ Get a pedaler, a little machine with a pair of bike pedals on a small stand. Put it under your desk and pedal while you work.

✔ Keep hand weights or resistance bands in your drawer, then take short breaks to bust a few strength-training moves. You'll work off some frustrations, too!

—MICHAEL ROIZEN, MD, CHIEF WELLNESS OFFICER AT THE CLEVELAND CLINIC AND CO-AUTHOR OF *YOU: THE OWNER'S MANUAL*

> **WHY IT WORKS** → Small breaks from butt-in-chair time can make a big health difference. In one Australian study, people who took more short, low-intensity breaks throughout the day—even just walking to the water fountain—were slimmer and trimmer and had lower blood sugar than long-haul desk jockeys. "That's super important, because uninterrupted sitting is a health threat all by itself," says Roizen. "It boosts your risk for abdominal fat, diabetes, heart disease, and some types of cancer."

MAKE IT EASY ON YOURSELF

You have to keep exercise fun, easy, and cheap. So I've started jumping rope, Hula Hooping, and boxing. Even though I live in California and love to surf and play tennis, frankly, it's nice to have things I can do anytime, anywhere."

—LISA MASTERSON, MD, OBSTETRICIAN/GYNECOLOGIST IN SANTA MONICA, CALIFORNIA, AND COHOST OF *THE DOCTORS*

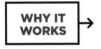 → Because it's doable. If you're among the millions missing out on shaping up, do what Masterson does: home workouts. In a recent national survey of 1,200 people, most of the 75% who said they exercise regularly stick with easy routines they can do on their own.

Don't get overwhelmed. Go for the minimum. Just 22 minutes a day of brisk walking plus two strength-training workouts a week—15 to 20 minutes each—is all you need to tone up your major muscle groups (arms, torso, legs). You can even do it in bite-size breaks if you need to: The CDC says it's fine to split exercise up into a couple of 10-minute mini sessions daily—say, spend half of it dancing to your favorite tunes in the living room and half using hand weights while you watch TV. Or do another thing Masterson does: Buy a Hula Hoop and get your wiggle on!

FIVE STICK-WITH-IT SECRETS

If you're among the countless adults (including some docs) who can always find something better to do than break a sweat, you've probably got a stack of barely used exercise clothes, a missing waistline, and a gym bag full of guilt. But even if "sign up for cool new kick-boxing class" will never appear on your to-do list, you can develop a regular workout habit with these five tricks. They harness your willpower, optimism, and pride.

1 **SET SMALL GOALS.** "Good intentions often lead to overly ambitious plans. Instead of promising yourself (again) that starting this morning, you'll exercise every day for the rest of your life, set a saner, more manageable goal. Say, aim for every other day this month. That's just 15 sessions during the next four weeks," says Roy F. Baumeister, PhD, psychologist at Florida State University and author of *Willpower: Rediscovering the Greatest Human Strength.*

WHY IT WORKS Walking 15 days a month will do you a ton of good. And if you aim for 15 but actually manage 20, you'll feel great about surpassing your goal.

2 **USE SOCIAL MEDIA.** Write down on each workout day whether or not you exercised—and keep your log online where friends or virtual fitness buddies can cheer you on or prod you to stick with it. Plenty of websites and apps can help you buddy up, including Fitness Buddy (fitnessbuddyapp.com) and the Nike+ running app (nike.com/nikeplus).

WHY IT WORKS Most of us do better when we're accountable to someone else.

3 **PICK A PEAK WILLPOWER HOUR.** Trying to force yourself to go for a jog after sitting through a boring presentation or redoing the family budget is always hard, even though you aren't physically tired. Schedule workouts for times when your stick-with-it powers haven't already been tested. Yes, this usually means in the morning.

WHY IT WORKS Tedious mental tasks like staying focused during a dull office meeting drain the same willpower reserves that exercise taps, Baumeister says.

4 **DON'T WATCH THE CLOCK.** "If you can get yourself to work out for even a few minutes one day, you're more likely to do it again the next day, and the next," says Suzanne Segerstrom, PhD, University of Kentucky psychologist and an expert on optimism.

WHY IT WORKS Starting any habit is the hardest part. Once you do, exercise habits get easier and easier to sustain.

5 **EXPECT SLIP-UPS.** You slept in, went to a birthday lunch, worked way too late to work out? No biggie. Just fit in 10 minutes somewhere, even if it means walking around the parking lot twice or marching in place while you watch *The Late Show*. Then remind yourself that tomorrow's another day, says Segerstrom.

WHY IT WORKS An optimistic outlook lets you see inevitable slip-ups not as deal breakers but as normal parts of reaching your goal.

THE ONLY WAY TO FIX BELLY FAT

I advise friends to do 150 minutes of exercise per week—that's just 22 minutes a day—but to make sure at least two or three of those days are for strength training.

—MARIA COLLAZO-CLAVELL, MD, ENDOCRINOLOGIST AT THE MAYO CLINIC, ROCHESTER, MINNESOTA

WHY IT WORKS → "Women are always surprised to learn that hormone-related weight gain, which starts happening in midlife, can be quite resistant to aerobics," says Collazo-Clavell. "Extra cardio won't hurt, but it's not what helps! You've got to alternate it with a few days of strength training."

10-SECOND SOLUTIONS

INSTANT INSPIRATION

Regular workouts help control weight, build sleek and sexy muscle, make you upbeat, keep your brain sharp, energize every inch of you, protect against oodles of serious health problems, and make you proud.

DEFINE "TOO SICK TO WORK OUT"

You have to let the flu or some other nasty bug run its course. Many people start pushing themselves as soon as they begin to feel a bit better—and then get knocked back down. I swear by the 72-hour rule: no workouts for at least three days after a fever breaks, and that's only if you're feeling much better. When you do go back, cut the intensity of your workout in half until all of your symptoms are gone.

—**IAN K. SMITH**, MD, FORMER COHOST OF *THE DOCTORS* AND *NEW YORK TIMES* BEST-SELLING AUTHOR OF *SUPER SHRED, SHRED, THE 4 DAY DIET, THE FAT SMASH DIET*, AND *EXTREME FAT SMASH DIET*

LEVERAGE PET POWER

If you're an animal lover, start making your dog walks increasingly active. It'll be good for both of you. Many docs know all about pet-induced motivation: I'll get home after work and feel tired, but our run together is the highlight of my dog's day. He'd be heartbroken if I skipped it!

—**ROY F. BAUMEISTER**, PHD, PSYCHOLOGIST AT FLORIDA STATE UNIVERSITY AND AUTHOR OF *WILLPOWER: REDISCOVERING THE GREATEST HUMAN STRENGTH*

GET YOUR KIDS MOVING, TOO

To help your kids get trimmer, fitter, and healthier, think play, not exercise. Before their mid-teens, kids' minds and bodies aren't ready for grown-up workouts. Long, intense, steady-state exercise is almost impossible for them to sustain and can even hurt their immature metabolic systems. Think fun bursts of activity instead.

For example, I worked with a mom who wanted her kids to go walking with her on a local track, but it bored the pants off them. However, when she started walking along the bayou instead, the kids had a ball—they could look for turtles and alligators and explore. After that, they loved walking there with her.

—**MELINDA S. SOTHERN**, PHD, PROFESSOR AT LOUISIANA STATE UNIVERSITY HEALTH SCIENCES CENTER IN NEW ORLEANS AND AUTHOR OF *TRIM KIDS: THE PROVEN 12-WEEK PLAN THAT HAS HELPED THOUSANDS OF CHILDREN ACHIEVE A HEALTHIER WEIGHT* AND *SAFE AND EFFECTIVE EXERCISE FOR OVERWEIGHT YOUTH*

WHY IT WORKS → "Kids are self-regulating when they play—they have intense bursts of activity, then quiet down, then become really active again," Sothern says. "Work with, not against, their natural rhythms and they'll happily run, jump, skip, and hop their way to better health." If you don't have a nearby bayou/park/creek, try bringing a box of balls, active games, and jump ropes to the local track or sports spot and let them play on the infield while you walk. Then get them to "help you" stretch as you cool down afterward. They'll be ready to go again soon.

BUILD FAMILY FITNESS HABITS

Motivating kids to be active without preaching or pushing isn't always easy. But making it fun, doing it regularly, and being a role model helps children develop lasting fitness habits on their own. When my daughter was little, she rode her bike alongside me while I ran. To celebrate her college graduation, we went hiking together on the Lycian Way in Turkey—roughly a 300-mile walk!

It's not just little kids. Parents have the power to influence teens' exercise habits, too. Having active fun together and supporting their interests by, say, driving them to sports practices or dance classes, talking up the coolness of being fit and strong, and staying fit themselves —even just by doing regular yard work or full-tilt housecleaning—are all factors that boost children's activity levels.

—CAROLYN BERNSTEIN MD, FAHS, ASSISTANT PROFESSOR OF NEUROLOGY AT THE HARVARD-AFFILIATED BRIGHAM AND WOMEN'S HOSPITAL IN BOSTON AND AUTHOR OF *THE MIGRAINE BRAIN*

 "In an intriguing study of 100 kids aged four to seven, what parents *do* turned out to make all the difference," says Bernstein. "Kids whose mothers worked out regularly were twice as active in their daily lives as kids whose parents rarely exercised. Kids with active fathers were three times more active. And those with two active parents were nearly six times more active! Similarly, British researchers have found that children with active parents are 50% more likely to be fit themselves than kids whose parents rarely leave the couch."

THE BEAT-BEAT-BEAT THAT BOOSTS MOTIVATION

TRY THIS: When you've reached your "cruising speed" in a steady-state workout, like running on a treadmill, pedaling a bike, or using an elliptical trainer, put on some music with a tempo that's in time with your movements. In research by Costas Karageorghis, PhD, reader in sport psychology at Brunel University London in the United Kingdom and a specialist in how music affects athletes and exercisers, exercisers worked out 15% longer before feeling exhausted and felt 15% better during their routine.

WHY IT WORKS → The tempo of exercise music could help you stay motivated—just ask any spin class or Zumba instructor. For music to get you revved up at the start of your workout, cue up tunes with a tempo of 130 to 140 beats per minute. Find the bpm of your favorite workout songs on websites such as www.songbpm.co, www.bpmdatabase.com. or www.jog.fm.

SMALL STEPS MATTER MOST

Often, what's standing in your way is . . . you. If you're trying to lose weight, for example, instead of focusing on your final far-off goal, just take one small step toward that goal *today*. For me, instead of planning a long workout every morning, I have a seven-minute routine that I *always* do.

—MEHMET OZ, MD, HOST OF THE AWARD-WINNING *DR. OZ SHOW* AND PROFESSOR OF SURGERY, COLUMBIA UNIVERSITY COLLEGE OF PHYSICIANS AND SURGEONS

WHY IT WORKS → "It's not an hour, it's seven minutes. For the rest of the day, I feel good that I did it, and that spurs me to make more good choices," says Oz.

ANSWERS TO
FITNESS IQ

1 **C.** Three out of four morning exercisers were still working out regularly a year later in one survey. But just half of lunchtime exercisers and a quarter of the evening group were still going strong. The simple reason: You're less likely to have schedule conflicts early in the day. *See page 126*.

2 **C.** A consistent routine that includes cardiovascular exercise (walking, swimming, taking an aerobics class, cycling, working out on an elliptical trainer) blasts calories and burns *overall* fat. But it takes strength training to help evaporate midlife belly fat! *See page 121*.

3 **C.** Home routines can be just as good as weight machines at building sleek, calorie-burning muscle, say fitness experts. That's great news if you don't have the time or budget for a gym membership or simply prefer to work out in the privacy of your own home. *See pages 117 and 127*.

4 **A.** Docs say it's wise to wait three days after a fever breaks before resuming your workouts. Even then, cut back on the intensity for a bit to avoid wearing yourself out. *See page 122*.

5 **C.** Before their teen years, kids aren't developmentally ready for long, steady-paced exercise—yep, that's the reason your seven-year-old complains on fitness walks and your 11-year-old would rather goof off. In contrast, bursts of activity are just right. Taking a critter-spotting nature walk, playing a ball game, or trying out a walking trail with "play" (exercise) equipment along the way satisfies their need for varied stop-and-go activity. When it's fun, they'll look forward to doing it again. *See page 123*.

6 **B.** Matching your workout music to your own heart rate makes you *want* to keep going, experts say. Use the easy formula to figure out your target heart rate for exercise, then find music with the same beats per minute online (there are sites that do just this) for a truly personalized soundtrack. *See page 125*.

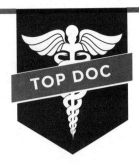

REMEMBER THESE FOUR RULES OF THE WORKOUT ROAD

We bet fitting in exercise finally seems doable after reading this chapter. Follow these five guidelines to create a plan that works for you:

1 **DON'T GO TO THE GYM.** At least not always. Working out at home—with resistance bands, a mini trampoline, a Hula Hoop, or just doing multiple flights of stairs—is a time-saving way to fit exercise in on a busy day. You won't waste precious minutes driving, parking, and changing in the locker room. And the results you can achieve are just as good.

2 **MAKE IT PERSONAL.** Choose activities you love. You'll feel more motivated and happier. A family bike ride, a walk with your very best friend, or a snappy Zumba class is a lot more fun than a half hour on the treadmill.

3 **SHORT IS BRILLIANT.** On days when exercise is one more stress or your schedule has only a tiny opening for a workout, exercise for just a few minutes. You may feel inspired to keep going once you get started. But even if you don't do more than six or seven minutes, you've burned a few calories, challenged your muscles, revved up your circulation, taken a quick mind/body break, and—yes!—maintained your exercise habit.

4 **WORK OUT AT WORK.** In addition to formal exercise, take short movement breaks every half hour or so when you're sitting at your desk. Extended sitting dials down your metabolism in ways that increase risk for heart disease, diabetes, and even some cancers—even for people who set aside dedicated exercise time.

5 **BUDDY UP.** Having set exercise dates with your partner, neighbor, office mate, or anyone else keeps you accountable (it's why one top doc gets up before dawn to go running). It's also more fun. And if you have kids, it sets a powerful example about the importance of being fit.

CHAPTER

8

ODD BUT NORMAL STUFF

IF YOU HAVE A PRETTY COMMON PROBLEM—from belly bloat to relentless bad breath—we've included doctors' advice, as well as the standard solutions and a few unusual ones, too. Docs know many of us do the same, going online to check out preventive strategies and popular treatments for everyday health issues, hoping they'll work.

Here's the thing: That's what this book and (especially this chapter) is all about! Providing doctor-sourced solutions for many kinds of common health problems—but also emphasizing clear "get professional help" guidelines when they're needed, because neither you nor physicians should try to treat anything serious on your own.

That said, you're about to find a bevy of tips about everything from "leaks" and gluten intolerance to helping doctor-shy guys get medical care. In the mix:

▶ What to do when stress freezes up your digestive system.

▶ The funny-provocative secret of avoiding vaginal infections— thank a top gynecologist for this one.

▶ A "cleansing" fad you should definitely skip.

▶ Favorite kitchen remedies from a top family physician.

▶ And a quick, simple home test if you love cheese, milk, and yogurt but think you're becoming lactose intolerant.

It all starts right here.

TEST YOUR
BODY QUIRKS KNOWLEDGE

Top docs often opt for simple solutions to non-emergency health concerns. While you might dash to the drugstore for a high-test mouthwash if your spouse says your breath is iffy, a top doc might just open the fridge. You might reach for a laxative if you've been irregular for a day or two, but a top doc might just drink more water, have some extra fruit, and take a walk. Are you as "no-nonsense" about day-to-day health maintenance as they are? Find out with this quiz.

1 If you suspect you're sensitive to gluten (a protein found in wheat and some other grains), the best thing to do is:

a. Switch to foods labeled "gluten-free."

b. Eat more fresh, unprocessed foods and a wider variety of grains.

c. See your doc for a test.

2 One surprising way to freshen bad breath is:

a. Chewing mint leaves

b. Eating yogurt

c. Rinsing your mouth with tea

3 Stress doesn't just make you jumpy. It can affect your intestinal tract by:

a. Making heartburn hurt more

b. Stalling out your digestion

c. Both

4 True or false: A "colonic" will cleanse your GI tract, promoting optimal health.

5 One surprising source of pesticides in your home is:

a. Your pet's flea-and-tick collar

b. Airborne chemicals drifting in from neighborhood yards or fields

c. Residue brought in on your shoes

6 Common kitchen staples that can help ease common health complaints include:

a. Frozen peas, honey, and onions

b. Blueberry jam and maple syrup

c. Crackers and spaghetti

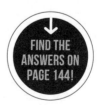

FIND THE ANSWERS ON PAGE 144!

KICK OFF YOUR UNDERWEAR

When I get home from work, I immediately change my clothes, which includes kicking off my undies entirely. I usually put on a pair of loose exercise pants, so there's no concern about embarrassing my children! And I certainly never wear underwear to bed.

I know women who are never out of their undies except in the shower. But wearing underwear 100% of the time traps moisture and body heat, which can increase the growth of bacteria in the genital area around the vagina, called the vulva. If you notice a not-fresh smell, usually the odor is coming from bacteria that grow after your vulva has been trapped in underwear for hours and hours.

The problem can be even worse in the winter, when women often wear panties, tights, or pantyhose and then snug jeans. Obviously, you don't want to have a Paris Hilton moment at work, so wear underwear during the day. But as soon as you get home, the underpants should come off. And no woman ever needs to wear them to bed.

—HILDA Y. HUTCHERSON, MD, PROFESSOR OF OBSTETRICS AND GYNECOLOGY AT COLUMBIA UNIVERSITY MEDICAL CENTER AND AUTHOR OF *WHAT YOUR MOTHER NEVER TOLD YOU ABOUT SEX AND PLEASURE*

 WHY IT WORKS → Tight clothing that can trap heat and moisture near your skin—pantyhose, body shapers, skinny jeans, leggings, dance clothes, yoga pants, and underwear—encourages bacteria, yeast infections, and vaginitis (swelling, irritation). Change out of these clothes as soon as possible when you get home or after a workout. Cotton underwear is usually a better choice than most stretchy synthetics. Although newer synthetics can be more breathable and dry faster.

SAY NO TO COLONICS

Friends often boast to me, "I just had a detoxing colonic!" because they think it's healthy, but I always say, "Don't follow that fad. The bacteria in our guts are there for a reason." In recent years, researchers are finding out more and more about what's called the "gut microbiome"—microorganisms that include trillions of bacteria. We used to think they didn't have much of a purpose aside from helping with vitamin absorption. But there's increasing evidence these bacteria play an important role in a wide range of problems, including obesity, diabetes, heart disease, and a number of immune and inflammatory conditions. So if you're washing them out, you could be losing bacteria your body needs for important functions.

Besides, I'm a gastroenterologist and do colonoscopies all the time, so I know our colons are usually very good at self-cleaning and flushing out toxins naturally. Most people just need to eat lots of veggies, fruit, and fiber to keep things working smoothly. So ditch the fruit juice in the morning and eat an orange or a grapefruit instead. That's one of the easiest ways to get more fiber. And stand by as scientists figure out how to improve health and combat illness by manipulating the microbiome using probiotics and diet.

—JONATHAN LAPOOK, MD, GASTROENTEROLOGIST AND CHIEF MEDICAL CORRESPONDENT FOR CBS NEWS

 Often promoted by fad-following celebrities and internet hucksters, colonics promise to purge toxins, infuse glowing good health, and resolve a laundry list of complaints, from constipation and allergies to pain.

But when Georgetown University Medical School researchers reviewed 20 colon-cleanse studies, they found little evidence of benefits—and problems ranging from cramping, bloating, and vomiting to electrolyte imbalances, kidney failure, and even death. While advocates claim the colon is home to toxic sludge deposits that exacerbate health issues, this idea was discredited decades ago by the American Medical Association. Instead, take LaPook's advice and eat plenty of satisfying, fiber-rich fruit, veggies, and whole grains. It's an alternative your pocketbook and your body will love.

AUTOMATE THE EASY STUFF

Life is a balance between change and constancy. Change keeps things interesting, but it's challenging. You can save energy for the tougher challenges if you make parts of your routine constant. For example, I like breakfast, but I also don't need much variety then. So I automatically have the same thing every day: yogurt and fruit. No decisions needed. It saves me time and energy for other tasks.

—**MEHMET OZ**, MD, HOST OF THE AWARD-WINNING *DR. OZ SHOW* AND PROFESSOR OF SURGERY, COLUMBIA UNIVERSITY COLLEGE OF PHYSICIANS AND SURGEONS

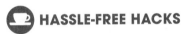 **HASSLE-FREE HACKS**

▶ **IN TERMS OF EVERYDAY HEALTH** with ongoing payoffs, think about two or three healthy steps you'd be happy to "automate"—to repeat every day and happily not give another thought to. It could be coming up with your own version of Oz's healthy breakfast—say, peanut butter and sliced bananas on whole-wheat toast. A daily dose of peanuts (and most nuts) lowers your risk of cancer, heart disease, and lung problems.

▶ **ANOTHER EXAMPLE:** walking the same two-mile route most mornings on autopilot. It's a no-brainer daily routine that slashes the threat of diabetes, heart attacks, and stroke.

▶ **AND/OR TRY CARVING OUT** five minutes after the dinner dishes are done to de-stress with a cup of chamomile tea. Soothing chronic stress helps you sidestep anxiety, insomnia, depression, and weight gain.

 There's a growing movement among prevention-minded health experts called "make the healthy choice the easy choice." It sounds like a no-brainer, but it's all about setting up your world so that health *is* automatic . . . because, say, you've stocked the fridge with your favorite hummus plus sliced carrots and peppers to dunk in for a healthy snack (instead of reaching for chips 'n' dip), stashed your favorite frozen fruit in the freezer for healthy smoothies, *and* made a standing walking date with a friend who's beyond reliable. When healthy choices are this easy, well-being is, too.

MAKE NICE TO YOUR MOUTH

I always say, only floss and brush the teeth you want to keep. Floss and brush them daily and you'll be rewarded with more than just a bright smile. Several studies have linked periodontal (gum) disease to heart disease. What's the connection? The thinking is that chronic gum disease causes chronic inflammation in your body, which in turn can cause swelling around the arteries.

—MICHAEL ROIZEN, MD, CHIEF WELLNESS OFFICER AT THE CLEVELAND CLINIC AND CO-AUTHOR OF *YOU: THE OWNER'S MANUAL*

WHY IT WORKS → "Your oral health has a major influence on the health of the rest of your body," Roizen explains. "The same bacteria that cause gum disease in your mouth can get into your bloodstream via infected gums and set off an immune reaction that can lead to heart disease and even stroke. Oh, and wrinkles, too!"

BE A LIAR

"Well, sort of. You can still be on a weight-loss plan without sacrificing your social life. I always tell clients to 'make it up' when it comes to food pushers (who you're not related to). You can decline, but if you find their pushing too aggressive, say you have an allergy. You'll feel more in control of the situation and you won't be worried about offending anyone or having to share your weight-loss goals with a full dinner table."

—JACLYN LONDON, MS, RD, GOOD HOUSEKEEPING NUTRITION DIRECTOR

GIVE YOURSELF SOME LOVE

The most important aspect of my self-care efforts is believing that I *deserve* to nurture myself—to eat well, exercise, dream, get a massage, or sometimes just curl up with a good book and do nothing. So many women take care of everyone else but themselves. Taking care of me gives me the energy to bring my best to the world.

But I also like to think about ways to make someone else's day. It's amazing what great energy this generates around me, and this in turn keeps my life joyous and makes me feel young and vibrant. It makes me more likely to get outdoors, connect with friends, and exercise—I love yoga, dancing, lifting weights, and jumping rope to rock 'n' roll. Enjoying life is the best outcome we can hope for!

—AVIVA ROMM, MD, CERTIFIED MIDWIFE, HERBALIST, AND AUTHOR OF *BOTANICAL MEDICINE FOR WOMEN'S HEALTH*, WINNER OF THE 2011 JAMES DUKE BOOK AWARD

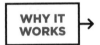

WHY IT WORKS → "I start every day with two essential practices: a few moments of gratitude and a healthy breakfast," Romm says, "although if I'm extra busy these might happen simultaneously! A grateful attitude keeps life in perspective, and a healthy breakfast keeps my blood sugar and mood steady all day and my metabolism humming. It also helps me make healthy food choices for the rest of the day."

CHILL OUT

A very busy attorney friend visited my family during a vacation in Hawaii. He was completely stressed out when he arrived, clutching a bottle of Tums, which he downed constantly for heartburn and stomach issues. But after relaxing at the beach all week, he ditched the Tums. He just didn't need them anymore!

Stress can wreak havoc on your stomach, because tension throughout the body can cause your digestive system to freeze up. If you're tightly wound all the time, the best OTC medication for stomach problems may be to chill out.

—PROFESSOR LIZ LIPSKI, PHD, CLINICAL NUTRITIONIST AND AUTHOR OF
DIGESTIVE WELLNESS

WHY IT WORKS → Your digestive system has a network of nerves that help coordinate the steps required to convert the burger you ate for lunch into fuel for energy and repairs. Researchers call this digestive nervous system the body's "second brain"—and it is exquisitely sensitive to stress. When life gets tough and you get tense, your digestion may slow down or completely stall. Stress can also make heartburn symptoms feel worse and increase irritating stomach acids.

Regular relaxation routines help and are far easier to come by than Hawaiian vacations. Six months of gentle yoga can soothe heartburn symptoms significantly, according to a recent study. And "gut-directed" hypnotherapy, cognitive behavioral therapy, and even simple techniques like progressive muscle relaxation (see page 67) can soothe digestive troubles like bloating, stomach pain, and even irritable bowel syndrome.

SPEAK UP ABOUT "LEAKS"

Urinary incontinence affects women of all ages—and men, too. But it's most common among pre- and post-menopausal women, especially those who have had children. It can be embarrassing and socially isolating, and many people hate to talk about it. But if it happens to you, promise yourself to bring it up at your next doctor appointment.

 Leaking can usually be treated, not just managed with absorbent pads. The options range from pelvic-floor exercises and bladder training to diet changes, weight loss, and, if needed, medication and/or surgery. Women shouldn't suffer in silence about this.

—**KEEHN HOSIER**, MD, OBSTETRICIAN-GYNECOLOGIST AT BROOKWOOD MEDICAL CENTER, BIRMINGHAM, ALABAMA

FLEA COLLARS AREN'T SO SMART

Adults who roughhouse and snuggle with pets wearing flea-and-tick collars contact up to 500 times the level of pesticides considered safe by the EPA. For children, the levels can be 1,000 times higher, according to a first-of-its-kind study by scientists at the Natural Resources Defense Council. (Pesticide poisoning can include nausea, vomiting, and difficulty breathing.)

The worst offenders are collars containing chemicals called (they're a mouthful) propoxur or tetrachlorvinphos, which kill pests by disrupting their nerve pathways. Many popular brands contain one of these substances, so check labels.

 Luckily, there are other options. "Pills that pets take seem to be safer," says Jerome Paulson, MD, director of the Mid-Atlantic Center for Children's Health and the Environment. Two common brands are Capstar and Program, which you can get from your vet or online for between $20 and $60. For other (often cheaper!) suggestions, check greenpaws.org.

BUILD A "HEALTHY YOU" TEAM

Surgeons don't perform surgery alone. We are surrounded by other doctors, nurses, and lab technicians who are better at their tasks than we could ever be. On my TV show, I also rely on an amazing staff with skill sets far beyond mine—everything I do is possible thanks to teamwork. Yet this is exactly where I see many of the women I talk to in the audience tripping up. They don't ask for help.

—MEHMET OZ, MD, HOST OF THE *DR. OZ SHOW* AND PROFESSOR OF SURGERY, COLUMBIA UNIVERSITY COLLEGE OF PHYSICIANS AND SURGEONS

 → It's smarter not to go it alone when it comes to reaching your health goals. Create a "healthy you" team to help you overcome obstacles. It could include family members, friends, and healthcare practitioners.

Start by thinking about what you need. Is it finding the time for exercise? Ask family members to take on some tasks that free up chunks of your time (running household errands on Saturday, making dinner twice a week—who cares if it's not perfect!). Or is it finding the motivation to exercise? Ask a friend to meet you for a regular walk or sign up for an exercise class together. Team up and you're both far more likely to work out regularly —and to reap the weight, health, and mood rewards.

A "healthy you" team is even more critical if you're managing a major health problem, like diabetes, high blood pressure, or heart disease. In one study, people with diabetes who formed teams with their doc and an expert or two—nutritionist, trainer—improved their blood sugar and felt more in control. Do it!

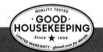

"Shedding for the wedding? Cut out starch (and other carbs) for 3 or 4 days prior to the big event. You'll drop water weight, since carbs are stored in the form of glycogen in your muscles (along with H_2O!), making you look leaner and less bloated."

—JACLYN LONDON, MS, RD, GOOD HOUSEKEEPING NUTRITION DIRECTOR

DON'T GUESS ABOUT GLUTEN INTOLERANCE

Many friends tell me, "I'm sure I'm allergic to gluten" if they have *any* gas, bloating, or diarrhea. But those symptoms can signal a lot of things, not just gluten intolerance.

Of course, if you've been diagnosed with celiac disease—meaning your body can't process gluten, the protein found in wheat, barley, and rye— that's obviously different. It can cause real health problems, including intestinal damage, and must be treated. But a lot of people have mild gluten tolerance. They don't need to go on a completely gluten-free diet, which is very restrictive.

I tell friends who are suddenly "sure" they're allergic to gluten to just try cutting back on foods that contain gluten rather than cutting them out completely. They're often able to tolerate a certain amount without any trouble.

—ROBERT BURAKOFF, MD, CLINICAL CHIEF OF GASTROENTEROLOGY AND DIRECTOR OF THE CENTER FOR DIGESTIVE HEALTH AT BRIGHAM AND WOMEN'S HOSPITAL IN BOSTON

WHY IT WORKS → Americans now spend more than $10 billion a year on pricey gluten-free foods, which have become almost fadlike. Some are super healthy, naturally gluten-free fruits, vegetables, and whole grains like quinoa and amaranth. But others are fatty, high-calorie, heavily processed foods like no-gluten pizza and Girl Scout cookies. It's great to eat lots of fresh, unprocessed foods . . . but do you need the other stuff, or even need to shun all gluten foods? Maybe not. Don't guess. Find out.

Your doctor can test you for celiac disease, a serious autoimmune disorder that an estimated 1.8 million Americans have—fortunately, less than 0.6% of the population. But up to 10 times that many—18 million more people—may be somewhat sensitive to wheat or gluten and experience everything from occasional headaches and fatigue to joint pain and digestive discomfort after eating offending foods. There's no test for mild to moderate intolerance, so work with your doctor to review your symptoms on and off gluten foods, and let that be your guide.

THREE NIFTY KITCHEN REMEDIES

No painkiller or icepacks on hand? No worries. Just use these home remedies from top family physician Reid B. Blackwelder, MD, of Kingsport, Tennessee, past president of the American Academy of Family Physicians.

1 **SOOTHE A MILD BURN WITH ONIONS.** Cut an onion in half and place it on the affected area until the pain subsides. The burn might be replaced by watering eyes, but that's a fair trade-off.

WHY IT WORKS "Onion juice contains sulfur compounds, quercetin, and other plant chemicals—the same ingredients in many over-the-counter burn treatments," Blackwelder explains.

2 **OPEN YOUR FREEZER TO RELIEVE A TENSION HEADACHE.** Grab a bag of frozen peas and hold it on the throbbing area for five to 10 minutes.

WHY IT WORKS "The cold constricts blood vessels, which eases pain, and frozen peas make a great, easily moldable, reusable ice pack," says Blackwelder.

3 **DEFLATE PUFFY EYES WITH TEA.** Apply tea bags soaked in cold water—black tea may be best, but any type will work.

WHY IT WORKS "Cool, wet things help decrease circulation and limit fluid buildup," Blackwelder says. "Plus the astringency of tea, due to its tannins, draws some fluid out as well."

THE CHUG TEST FOR LACTOSE INTOLERANCE

If a friend says she has too much gas, a churning tummy, and is constantly running to the bathroom, her next sentence is predictable: "Could dairy be the culprit?" To find out fast, I recommend this dairy challenge test: Drink a whole quart of low-fat milk in 15 to 30 minutes.

If you can down this amount and not get gas, bloating, and diarrhea, then you're probably fine. Many doctors recommend a slower option: cutting out dairy products for 10 days. If your symptoms ease up, you're likely lactose intolerant. But if you want to know *now*, the chug test will give you a good indication.

—BRIAN E. LACY, MD, PROFESSOR OF MEDICINE AND SECTION CHIEF OF GASTROENTEROLOGY AND HEPATOLOGY AT DARTMOUTH-HITCHCOCK MEDICAL CENTER, LEBANON, NEW HAMPSHIRE

WHY IT WORKS → Many people *are* lactose intolerant, and its symptoms—belly pain, nausea, and other digestive woes—can appear out of nowhere. You can develop lactose intolerance in your 30s or 40s or later; after surgery, chemotherapy, or taking penicillin; during pregnancy; or if you simply haven't had dairy products for a long time. That's when symptoms can be most confusing.

After early childhood, more than 60% of us don't produce enough of the enzyme lactase to fully break down lactose, the sugar in milk. Rates are highest among people of Native American, African, Asian, and Caribbean descent.

If you are lactose intolerant but you enjoy dairy foods and/or rely on them to keep your calcium intake high, try taking a lactase supplement (it's the digestive enzyme you're now missing) or drinking lactose-free milk. Either or both will likely help.

10-SECOND SOLUTIONS

QUICK FIX FOR BELLY BLOAT

Friends are constantly saying to me, "Ugh, I feel so bloated and my stomach's sticking out." I tell them—nicely!—to get moving. Research shows that physical activity can help, well, move gas out. Holding it in doesn't just make your tummy look distended; it's also plain uncomfortable. Exercise makes you look slimmer *and* feel better.

—**GAIL HECHT**, MD, DIVISION DIRECTOR OF GASTROENTEROLOGY AT LOYOLA UNIVERSITY MEDICAL CENTER, MAYWOOD, ILLINOIS

IFFY BREATH? GRAB A YOGURT

Enjoying six ounces of yogurt daily reduces levels of hydrogen sulfide—yep, that rotten-egg smell—produced by smelly mouth bacteria. Why isn't exactly clear, but it works. Don't like yogurt? "Almost any milk product or food that contains live cultures will likely have the same effect," says Robert Meltzer, MD, gastroenterologist and attending physician at Lenox Hill Hospital, New York City.

BOOK HIS AND HERS CHECKUPS

Worried that the man in your life is missing out on health checks and care? Schedule joint checkups. "Women are used to going to doctors regularly and can often get guys to go with them. The goal is helping men get the regular care that *prevents* major health problems or catches them early," says Mark A. Moyad, MD, MPH, preventive and alternative medicine expert affiliated with the University of Michigan Medical Center's Department of Urology.

NO, YOU'RE PROBABLY NOT IRREGULAR!

Whenever friends ask me if it's a problem if they don't go to the bathroom like clockwork, I tell them that the healthy number of bowel movements ranges from fewer than three per day to more than three per week. And yes, I understand it if you think we researchers who track these things probably have too much time on our hands!

But my point is, as long as you don't have bloating, constipation, or discomfort between "drop-offs," don't panic.

—WILLIAM D. CHEY, MD, PROFESSOR OF MEDICINE AND DIRECTOR OF THE GI PHYSIOLOGY LABORATORY, UNIVERSITY OF MICHIGAN HEALTH SYSTEM, ANN ARBOR

Lots of Americans think they're constipated, but a definitive review by the University of Michigan concluded that only about 12 to 19% of us get blocked up with any regularity.

One of the best ways to stay regular is simply by bumping up the fiber in your diet.

WHY IT WORKS → Getting at least 20 grams a day—the amount in a serving of high-fiber cereal, ½ cup of beans, two slices of whole-grain bread, and a couple of servings of fruit and veggies—cuts your risk for constipation almost in half. Wash it down with water to keep everything moving in the right direction.

Then take a walk. In a Harvard study, women who ate plenty of fiber and exercised daily cut constipation odds by almost 70%. Need more help? Skip laxatives and go the old-fashioned route: munch a prune (dried plum) or sip prune juice. This fruit has a natural laxative action—so be prudent. Eating too many may cause cramping, bloating, or diarrhea.

ANSWERS TO
BODY QUIRKS KNOWLEDGE

1 **B.** Up to 18 million Americans may be somewhat sensitive to gluten or other proteins in wheat and a few other grains, but there's no medical test yet for mild or moderate gluten intolerance. If you think gluten's bothering you, top docs advise **(a)** eating more nutritious, unprocessed foods that are naturally gluten-free, like fruit, vegetables, and nongluten grains; **(b)** limiting but not eliminating wheat and other glutinous grains to see if that helps you; **(c)** avoiding the glut of heavily processed gluten-free foods like pizza, ice cream, cookies, and chips—they're no healthier than any heavily processed foods. *See page 139.*

2 **B.** The live, active cultures in several yogurt brands (check labels) help keep mouth bacteria responsible for bad breath in line—perhaps by reducing acidity in your throat and esophagus. It's a delicious way to keep a lid on halitosis! *See page 142.*

3 **C.** You've probably heard that stress exacerbates heartburn, but did you know it can toss a monkey wrench into the nerve signals that choreograph digestion? Relaxation routines are the best remedy, top digestion experts say. *See page 136.*

4 **FALSE.** Colon "cleanses" are expensive and unnecessary (your digestive system excels at housekeeping), and could cause harm. In one big study, researchers recently found that colonics can cause problems ranging from cramping, bloating, and vomiting to electrolyte imbalances, kidney failure, and even death. A much better idea: Eat plenty of fruit and whole grains. *See page 132.*

5 **A.** It's always a good idea to avoid pesticides, and that includes pet flea-and-tick collars. They could expose your family to between 500 and 1,000 times the safe levels of pesticides set by the EPA. Instead, consider pest-fighting pills for pets. *See page 137.*

6 **A.** Top docs grab what works— frozen peas to ease a tension headache, a sliced onion to soothe minor burns, damp tea bags to shrink under-eye puffiness. You'll be a master of kitchen remedies, too, after reading this chapter! *See page 140.*

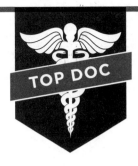

TOP DOC

REMEMBER THESE FIVE TIPS FOR DEALING WITH BODY ODDITIES

The top-doc approach to everyday health can be summed up in these five no-nonsense rules. Use them to guide decisions about your own well-being.

1 KEEP IT SIMPLE AND NATURAL. For truly small health concerns—minor skin irritations, bad breath, occasional constipation—turn first to sound home remedies that use stuff that's likely already in your kitchen. You'll save money and sidestep potential side effects of drugstore treatments.

2 APPROACH FOOD SENSITIVITIES WITH COMMON SENSE. You may have become intolerant to gluten or lactose—millions of people are—but don't guess. Do one of the self-checks in this chapter before you cut out important food groups and spend big bucks on special diets.

3 KNOW WHEN TO SEE THE DOC. Don't suffer in silence with ongoing health problems, whether it's occasional "leaks," persistent digestive issues, or something else. And if a man in your life is constantly putting off medical checkups, book a double appointment. Be creative and proactive as well as practical when it comes to everyday health care.

4 LITTLE THINGS MAKE A DIFFERENCE. One top doc cuts her risk for "down there" smells and infections by taking off her underwear as soon as she gets home from work. Another always looks for little ways to make someone else's day healthier and happier, which is contagious—it inevitably improves her own, too. Small, positive steps today add up to healthier tomorrows.

5 STEER CLEAR OF EXTREMES. Detoxing colonics, unusual supplements, and weird diets that promise to "fix" your health rarely do. Top docs draw a line between safe DIY strategies and crazy stuff that could cause harm. If it sounds crazy or scary, it probably is. Skip it.

RELIEF WHEN IT HURTS

T'S NOT JUST THE FRAMED DIPLOMA OR THE YEARS OF TRAINING that make so many top docs experts at preventing and relieving aches and pains. It's also because their know-how is often coupled with plenty of personal experience.

Case in point: In an eye-opening survey of 576 neurologists who specialize in headaches, the stunning number above—75%—had endured the blinding pain of migraines. In fact, the survey group suspects that living with big headaches likely inspired many of the docs to specialize in treating this debilitating pain, which adds an extra dose of compassion and urgency to their care.

Top docs usually don't reveal their own experiences with pain, injury, and illness to their patients—or the media. Chalk it up to professionalism, a sense of dignity, or a need to seem strong and be reassuring. As one migraine survey author told the *Chicago Tribune*, "We're pretty secretive about our migraines, but every one of us has our own way of coping." In this chapter, top docs reveal the tips, tricks, and strategies they use when facing these all-too-human moments, and their advice for patients. Among the experts who talked candidly about what they do and why:

▶ A headache doc who has—finally—learned how to defuse her own migraines.

▶ An outdoors-loving researcher who has devoted his life to helping others avoid the tiny, menacing ticks that spread Lyme disease and other painful infections.

▶ A top preparedness team who save lives with their ready-for-anything first aid kits.

▶ A burn-prevention expert who always practices what he preaches.

▶ There's plenty you can learn from what they do when something hurts . . . or threatens to.

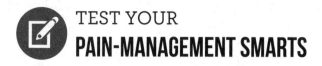

TEST YOUR
PAIN-MANAGEMENT SMARTS

Docs don't have time for pain—and neither do you. You might think they'd reach for a stash of pain pills, but top docs prefer to go with nondrug solutions whenever possible. They reserve meds for conditions that truly need them, like a full-blown migraine. The trick is to know which basic remedies work best for non-emergency aches and pains, and when to turn to something stronger. Test your knowledge with this quiz, then get the details ahead.

1 **One fixable source of tension headaches is:**

a. Doing your income taxes

b. Unconsciously clenching your jaw

c. Constantly twirling your hair

2 **You can prevent painful infections in cuts and scrapes by:**

a. Immediately slathering on a germ-fighting ointment and a bandage

b. Flushing out the cut or scrape with alcohol

c. Washing the area with water and mild soap or a saline solution

3 **If you find a tick on your body— putting you at risk for painful Lyme disease and other tick- borne illnesses—treat it by:**

a. Globbing on petroleum jelly to suffocate it

b. Touching it with a hot match to stun or kill it

c. Using pointy tweezers to pull it out

4 **If you're prone to migraines, two underestimated ways to deter these intense headaches are:**

a. Drinking lots of water and getting plenty of sleep

b. Drinking tea twice a day

c. Taking a warm bath every morning and night

5 **True or false:** The best way to handle a muscle strain is to slowly "walk it off."

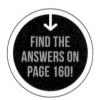

FIND THE ANSWERS ON PAGE 160!

GET ON-THE-SPOT BACK PAIN RELIEF

One great trick I use when a back muscle is tense is to roll a small towel into a ball, lie flat on the floor, and place it directly under the part of my back that hurts. Then I put my hands on my belly and just relax.

—MICHAEL ROIZEN, MD, CHIEF WELLNESS OFFICER AT THE CLEVELAND CLINIC AND CO-AUTHOR OF *YOU: THE OWNER'S MANUAL*

If that's not enough to take the edge off the ache, try everyday anti-inflammatories like naproxen (Aleve) and ibuprofen (Advil, Motrin). Why not go for something stronger? A landmark report on back pain treatments from the American College of Physicians and the American Pain Society found that these ordinary meds offered "moderate" benefit. But prescription painkillers—which cost more and can have more serious side effects—also came in as "moderate."

WHY IT WORKS → Research shows that most back pain gets better without heavy-duty painkillers or surgery. To relax tight muscles fast, try the tennis ball tip on page 83. Afterward, do some gentle stretching or yoga. Why? The same pain report found that exercise therapy and yoga routines that emphasize stretching and body control are the best workouts for back pain sufferers.

Just don't "stretch through" or "push beyond" anything painful. If pain persists, ask your doctor for a referral to a physical therapist, who will show you how to exercise safely and get the most out of it.

Need more help? Consider seeing a chiropractor. A definitive review of 39 randomized, controlled studies rated chiropractic treatments for lower back pain about on par with pain meds or exercise.

MAKE THE MOST OF MIGRAINE TREATMENTS

Doctors aren't immune to illnesses, though sometimes patients think we are. I'm a migraine sufferer. I needed preventive medications in the past, but fortunately my migraines have become less frequent and less severe. But they still happen. When they do, I know I need to take anti-migraine medication early for the best results.

But it's really important not to overdo it. Using prescription anti-migraine drugs or pain medication more than 10 days a month can lead to medication overuse headaches. These drugs lower your migraine threshold over time. It's as if you're teaching brain cells to become pain cells. Work with your doctor if this is happening to you.

—**CHRISTINA PETERSON**, MD, DIRECTOR OF THE OREGON HEADACHE CLINIC IN CLACKAMAS, OREGON, AND AUTHOR OF *THE WOMEN'S MIGRAINE SURVIVAL GUIDE*

"One of the things that helps me prevent a migraine is staying hydrated," Peterson says. "I make sure I drink water or tea throughout the day. I also take a magnesium supplement that acts to suppress migraines."

Good basic self-care can make a difference, too. In a study of women with daily or near-daily migraines, those who adopted a strict eight-hours-a-night sleep schedule enjoyed a 29% drop in migraine frequency and a 40% drop in pain.

While about 40% of the 32 million Americans who get migraines could get relief with the right medicine, two out of three don't, found one study. Your migraines may not be frequent or severe enough to warrant regular use of a preventive drug, but using the right one can stop a migraine in its tracks.

SIDESTEP PAINFUL LYME DISEASE

Whenever I've been outdoors in tick habitat, and at least once a day anyway, I check myself for ticks as soon as possible after coming indoors, being careful not to overlook the out-of-the-way spots where ticks often attach.

While ticks can attach themselves any place on your body, they all crawl upward until they meet resistance, usually stopping to bite in areas where clothing or skin folds slow their upward crawl—often below the belt, like the backs of knees; around underwear lines, waistbands, and bra straps; but also the backs of arms, armpits, and hairline, and behind ears. You've just got to lean over and look, and be creative with mirrors. Once they've dug in, they won't wash off or drown in the shower, so check your entire body while naked.

To remove a tick, don't cover it with petroleum jelly or touch a hot match to it. Those folk legends are not safe and could increase disease risk. Wipe the tick and the skin around it with a swab soaked in alcohol, then use pointy tweezers to carefully pull out the tick. Clean the area with more alcohol, an iodine scrub, or soap and water.

—**THOMAS MATHER**, PHD, ENTOMOLOGY PROFESSOR AT THE UNIVERSITY OF RHODE ISLAND AND DIRECTOR OF THE SCHOOL'S CENTER FOR VECTOR-BORNE DISEASE AND TICKENCOUNTER RESOURCE CENTER

 "It generally takes 24 hours for a nymph stage blacklegged tick and 48 hours for an adult to transmit Lyme disease and some of the other infections they carry to a human host," Mather says. "If you suspect a tick has been on you for that long and you're concerned about infection, you can submit a picture of the tick to assess its riskiness (www.tickencounter.org/tickspotters) and also save the tick in a bottle or sealed plastic bag and have it tested for disease."

PREVENT A BURN

A bad burn is one of the most painful injuries anyone can get, and it can easily happen at home. In our kitchen, the cooktop is on an island. I'm constantly removing cookbooks, recipes, and mail left near the cooking surface. If people gather around when I cook, I'm vigilant about keeping them from standing too close.

Cooking is the leading cause of home fires (45%) and home fire injuries (42%). Knowing how to lower the danger of a kitchen fire and what to do if you have one could prevent a severe, painful burn or even save your life, your family's lives, and your home. The commonsense rules below help. If your children are old enough to cook, teach them to follow the rules, too.

—**ROBERT COLE**, PHD, PRESIDENT OF COMMUNITY HEALTH STRATEGIES AND ASSOCIATE PROFESSOR OF CLINICAL NURSING, UNIVERSITY OF ROCHESTER MEDICAL CENTER, ROCHESTER, NEW YORK

AVOID MISTAKES

✔ Don't cook when you're tired or have been drinking.

✔ When you're frying, grilling, or broiling, don't leave the kitchen or grill for even a moment without turning off the burners.

✔ Check slow-cooking food regularly; use a timer to remind you.

✔ Keep anything that can catch fire—oven mitts, wooden utensils, food packaging, dish towels—away from the stovetop.

✔ Wear short or snug sleeves when cooking. Loose clothing can catch fire if it comes in contact with a burner.

| WHAT TO DO | → | **KITCHEN ACCIDENTS HAPPEN. FOLLOW THESE STEPS IF A FIRE STARTS:** |

▶ Keep a lid nearby to smother small grease fires. If one flares up anyway, slide the lid over the pan and turn off the stove. Leave the pan covered until it's completely cool.

▶ For an oven fire, turn off the heat and keep the door closed.

▶ If these steps don't contain the fire immediately, get out! When you leave, close the door of your home behind you.

▶ Call 911 *after* you're outside.

USE TEA TO CALM CRAMPS

Something I always did to relieve menstrual cramps was to drink red raspberry leaf tea. It's a traditional herbal remedy that relaxes the muscles of the uterus. It helped me.

Brew a cup by simmering a small handful of dried or fresh leaves in two cups of boiling water for a minute or two. Then turn off the heat and let the tea steep for about 10 minutes. Strain and sip. Just don't expect a blast of raspberry! It tastes like ordinary black tea.

—**HILDA Y. HUTCHERSON**, MD, PROFESSOR OF OBSTETRICS AND GYNECOLOGY AT COLUMBIA UNIVERSITY MEDICAL CENTER AND AUTHOR OF *WHAT YOUR MOTHER NEVER TOLD YOU ABOUT SEX AND PLEASURE*

 → "Rich in vitamins and minerals, this Native American herb has been used for centuries. Modern experts say compounds in red raspberry leaves may have a relaxing effect on blood vessels and smooth muscle tissue," says Hutcherson. "It also helps ease nausea. Herbalists who specialize in women's health credit the tea's effects to an alkaloid called fragrine."

Other natural strategies that may help prevent menstrual cramps include quitting smoking, cutting back on alcohol, and eating more fiber-rich fruits, vegetables, and whole grains. In a Japanese study of 276 women, the biggest fiber eaters had the least menstrual pain. Simply hanging in helps, too: Menstrual cramps tend to back off as you get older.

WHAT'S IN A *GREAT* FIRST AID KIT

Every home and car should have a better-than-basic first aid kit. You never know what you'll need or when. I've used mine for everything from kitchen cuts to a car accident I came across when I was on the road. The well-dressed kit includes everything on the list below.

—AMY ALTON, ARNP, CO-AUTHOR OF *THE SURVIVAL MEDICINE HANDBOOK* AND CO-FOUNDER OF THE SURVIVAL MEDICINE WEBSITE

BANDAGES AND DRESSINGS

ADHESIVE AND BUTTERFLY BANDAGES for minor cuts and scrapes

STERILE GAUZE PADS (4 x 4 inches)

LARGE WOUND DRESSINGS (9 x 5 inches or bigger) to cover severe cuts and absorb bleeding

NONSTICK DRESSINGS (like Telfa) to cover burns

ADHESIVE TAPE to secure dressings

BLISTER DRESSINGS like moleskin for sports and hiking

ROLL BANDAGES to wrap around and support a skin dressing

SCISSORS to cut through clothing so you can reach a wound without moving the injury

CUTS, BITES, AND BURNS

BURN RELIEF GELS to soothe pain

STING RELIEF PADS for insect bites

TWEEZERS AND NEEDLES to remove splinters or ticks and drain small abscesses

ANTIBIOTIC CREAM to help prevent infections in minor wounds

1% HYDROCORTISONE CREAM to decrease inflammation

ALCOHOL OR BETADINE PADS for disinfection

STRAINS AND SPRAINS

A DISPOSABLE COLD PACK to minimize swelling from sprains and other injuries

ELASTIC BANDAGES to support sprains

A TRIANGULAR BANDAGE that looks like a gauze bandanna; used with safety pins, it forms a sling for injured arms; in a pinch, it can serve as a tourniquet

SPLINTS to immobilize sprains and other injuries

MISCELLANEOUS

NONLATEX (NITRILE) GLOVES to protect both you and patients from infection; nitrile won't cause reactions in people allergic to latex

ORAL ANTIHISTAMINE, such as Benadryl, for allergic reactions

THERMOMETER to check for fevers

ACETAMINOPHEN, ASPIRIN, AND/ OR IBUPROFEN for pain and fever

FIRST AID BOOK for things you're unsure of—the American Red Cross guide is a classic

HOW TO STOP BLEEDING—FAST

Some years ago, an elderly neighbor fainted and fell, and I was called to help. She had a nasty gash on her thigh, and I needed to stop the bleeding quickly. Here's what to do if this ever happens to you:

The core treatment for bleeding wounds is simple: direct pressure, immediately. So if possible, have someone else call emergency services while you tend to the injury. Put on sterile gloves if they're available, or (more likely) use gauze bandages or a clean cloth to form a barrier between germ-laden hands and the injury. Apply direct pressure with your hands, then elevate the injured area above the level of the heart to slow the bleeding.

—JOSEPH ALTON, MD, RETIRED SURGEON, MEDICAL PREPAREDNESS EXPERT, AND CO-AUTHOR OF *THE SURVIVAL MEDICINE HANDBOOK*

> **WHAT HELPS** →

"If the bleeding's severe and direct pressure isn't enough, improvise a tourniquet with a belt or bandanna," says Alton.

"If there's an emergency dispatcher on the phone, ask for guidance in applying it. When help arrives, tell them what time the tourniquet was applied. Tissue damage can occur if it's left on too long."

HOW TO SELECT A FIRST AID KIT

"We recommend selecting one that has clearly labeled packets filled with items and instructions for common problems: cuts and scrapes, bleeding, wounds, burns, blisters, stings, splinters, sprains and strains, shock, CPR, and headaches and other pain. The items' expiration dates should be checked once a year and items restocked as needed. "

—BIRNUR ARAL, PHD, DIRECTOR, GOOD HOUSEKEEPING HEALTH, BEAUTY AND ENVIRONMENTAL SCIENCES LAB

10-SECOND SOLUTIONS

TENSION HEADACHE TAMER

While doctors aren't sure why we do it, clenching our teeth is a common response to stress. But it strains the big, powerful muscle that connects your jaw to your temples, and intense clenching can trigger a tension headache.

If this happens, the New England Center for Headache in Stamford, Connecticut, recommends you rest a pencil between your teeth—don't bite down. This relaxes your jaw muscles, eradicating tension and reducing pain. Note: This remedy only works for tension headaches, not migraines or sinus pressure

DON'T PUT UP WITH PAIN

An acquaintance was suffering from severe abdominal pain, unlike menstrual cramps. Her ob/gyn could not find the cause and effectively said, "There's nothing more I can do." She called me and said, "Jackie, my whole life is starting to center around this pain!" She'd already had her appendix taken out, so I suggested she see a different gynecologist immediately. She was diagnosed with endometriosis and had to have surgery.

Never ignore intense pain. If a doctor ever says or implies, "Live with the pain, dear," find another doctor.

—JACQUELINE WOLF, MD, GASTROENTEROLOGIST AT BETH ISRAEL DEACONESS MEDICAL CENTER IN BOSTON AND ASSOCIATE PROFESSOR OF MEDICINE AT HARVARD UNIVERSITY

DON'T SHRUG OFF MUSCLE STRAINS

Pulled a muscle trying out a new boot-camp workout or playing pick-up basketball? Make the ache short-lived with RICE, a tried-and-true method top docs swear by.

REST the injured body part.

ICE it for 20 minutes every three to four hours.

COMPRESS the injury with an elastic bandage.

ELEVATE the hurt area above your heart (say, by propping it on a pillow).

Do this for 48 hours. Your pain and swelling should start to subside. If not, see your doctor or go to the ER—especially if you can't bear weight, have significant bone or joint tenderness, or have severe swelling or an obvious deformity. Ignoring pain is never a good idea!

—**TRAVIS STORK**, MD, EMERGENCY MEDICINE PHYSICIAN AND HOST OF THE EMMY AWARD-WINNING DAYTIME SHOW *THE DOCTORS*

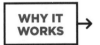 → The RICE formula works on several fronts to jumpstart healing. *Rest* keeps you from further injuring a strained muscle that needs inactivity to mend. *Ice* discourages inflammation—painful swelling is your body's way of making you stop using a hurt ankle or sore tennis elbow, but it can last unnecessarily long. Be careful not to apply ice directly to your skin. *Compression* and *elevation* also help limit swelling. Apply this strategy for the first two days; after that, gentle movement is often recommended to help you stay flexible. But check with your doc first; not all strains are the same.

CLEAN CUTS THE RIGHT WAY

A lot of people don't know how to treat a fresh cut. Instead of slapping on a bandage, which could trap bacteria inside, run to the nearest sink, spread the wound open, and wash it well to get as much germy junk out as possible.

When you're cleaning it, put nothing on the cut that you wouldn't put in your eye—water, mild soap, and saline are fine. Wash the skin around the wound, too. Then add a bandage if you like. But don't cover up a puncture wound. Leave it open and soak it in warm, soapy water two to three times daily for four or five days to keep it clean.

—MICHAEL ROIZEN, MD, CHIEF WELLNESS OFFICER AT THE CLEVELAND CLINIC; CO-AUTHOR OF *YOU: THE OWNER'S MANUAL*

> **WHAT HELPS** → Most small cuts and scrapes stop bleeding naturally in a few minutes and do fine with everyday products. But if bleeding continues, press a clean gauze pad over the cut firmly but gently. If it doesn't stop after 20 minutes or continues to soak through the bandage, call your doctor.

Also call your doc if a cut is large, deep, or jagged; is on your face; contains dirt you can't remove; starts oozing whitish-gray goop; or continues to look red and irritated, or if the redness gets worse. Infections of all types are becoming increasingly tricky to treat because so many bacteria are now antibiotic-resistant. You need professional help.

THE SMARTEST WAY TO SOOTHE A SUNBURN

Way back when I was a kid, sun lotions were designed to encourage tanning, not protect you from the sun. As a result, I got a severe second-degree burn over most of my back and arms when I was eight years old. Other than anesthetic sprays, not much helped. My parents thought they were doing me a favor by peeling off loose skin and popping blisters. Big mistake. It took me a month to heal.

Sunscreens today provide amazing protection, but burns still happen. If you or someone you love ever gets badly sunburned, here's a better way to treat it . . .

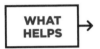 First-degree burns are superficial, affecting only the skin's outer layer (the epidermis). Your skin becomes warm and dry, and looks and feels mildly burned. For relief, place cool moist cloths on the area and start taking an anti-inflammatory, such as ibuprofen. Gently applying aloe vera or zinc oxide cream will also help. Discomfort will subside after 24 hours or so.

Second-degree burns become moist, weepy, and develop blisters. These deeper burns reach the skin's underlayer (the dermis). Run cool water over the area, then apply a moist protective dressing, like Spenco Second Skin. Anesthetic ointments and pain meds will help, and a silver-based burn cream, such as Silvadene, or antibiotic ointments will help prevent infections.

Third-degree burns are the most severe and should be treated as an emergency. Cover the area with a cool, moist dressing or cloth (do not use ice) and get professional help. You should also get emergency help for second-degree burns larger than three inches across that are on your face, hands, feet, face, groin, buttocks, or a major joint. Ditto for first-degree burns that cover a large portion of any of these extra-vulnerable areas.

—**JOSEPH ALTON**, MD, RETIRED SURGEON, MEDICAL PREPAREDNESS EXPERT, AND CO-AUTHOR OF *THE SURVIVAL MEDICINE HANDBOOK*

ANSWERS TO
PAIN-MANAGEMENT SMARTS

1 **B.** Clenching the large muscles that move your jaw is a common response to stress—you may be doing it right now and not even realize it. Tension there can slowly tighten other muscles in your neck and face, affecting nerves and triggering a bad headache. Easy solution: Gently hold a pencil between your teeth; this keeps those muscles loose. *See page 156.*

2 **C.** Cleaning cuts and scrapes with soap and water or saline solution—not alcohol—is step one in helping them heal well and quickly. Afterward, you can use an antibiotic ointment and bandage, but leave deep cuts or puncture wounds uncovered and clean them several times a day. *See page 158.*

3 **C.** Clean the area with alcohol, then remove the tick with tweezers. Killing it with a hot match or petroleum jelly is ineffective. You want this insect *out*, now, without hurting yourself in the bargain. Be sure to check favorite tick hiding spots after you've been outdoors, like the back of your knees, behind your ears, at your waistline. *See page 151.*

4 **A.** You can help cut the frequency and intensity of migraine headaches significantly by regularly getting plenty of sleep (8 hours every night according to one study) and drinking plenty of water to stay hydrated. You may still need medications to prevent or treat this head pain, but smart lifestyle steps should be a key part of your "stop pain before it starts" migraine strategy. *See page 150.*

5 **FALSE.** If you've pulled a muscle—gardening, moving furniture, playing sports, or dancing at your niece's wedding—baby that injury. Best strategy: rest, ice, compression with an elastic bandage, and then elevating the injured muscle. Do this for 48 hours. If pain doesn't subside, see your doc. *See page 157.*

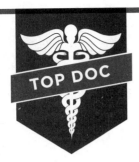

TOP DOC

REMEMBER THESE FIVE PAIN-STOPPING STEPS

Whether you're living with recurring pain or just want a better way to subdue occasional ouches and aches, top docs have the answers. Follow these rules of thumb:

1 START WITH SELF-CARE FOR SORE BACKS. Research shows that most back pain gets better without heavy-duty painkillers or surgery. That's important news for the one in four Americans living with this common—and often debilitating—ache. Over-the-counter pain relievers, gentle yoga and stretching (talk with your doc if pain is too severe for these), physical therapy, and spinal manipulation by a chiropractor can all help.

2 TAKE CONTROL OF HEADACHE TRIGGERS. If you're among the more than one in six Americans who get severe headaches and painful migraines, it's important to find and conquer everyday triggers so you can reduce their frequency and intensity. Once you do, you may need fewer or less potent drugs to handle the headaches you still get.

3 HAVE THE FIRST AID SUPPLIES AND SAVVY YOU NEED. Do you remember the best infection-fighting way to clean a cut? Soap and water—and lots of it. To stop bleeding? Fast, steady pressure. To soothe a sunburn? Cool compresses, ibuprofen, aloe vera cream. Refresh yourself on this chapter's advice *and* get a good first aid guide or phone app. Then stash emergency first aid kits in your car and at home.

4 BE SMART ABOUT PREVENTING PAINFUL INJURIES. Like a top doc, you now know how to spot and remove infectious ticks, put out sudden kitchen fires that cause painful burns, and much more. Use their advice and your new know-how to protect yourself and your family.

5 DON'T HESITATE TO GET HELP. While there's plenty you can do to prevent and ease pain, don't wait if you or a loved one needs medical assistance. Severe burns, deep wounds, intense pain, a cut that won't stop bleeding . . . all merit a call to the doctor pronto, or perhaps a trip to the ER or dialing 911.

CHAPTER 10

DON'T GET HEART DISEASE

HEART DISEASE IS AMERICA'S LEADING CAUSE OF DEATH (killing 380,000 people annually—a number that rises to over 700,000 a year if you include strokes and other cardiovascular "events"). What do MDs advise their patients to do to avoid it? It's all about paying attention to the details.

MAINTAIN HEALTHY CHOLESTEROL LEVELS, avoiding dangerously high total cholesterol of 240 or above, versus 10% of American men aged 60 and older.

AVOID HIGH BLOOD PRESSURE, the silent killer raging in the arteries of 33% of Americans.

EAT MORE FRUITS AND VEGETABLES and maintain a healthier weight—factors that slash your risk for developing high blood pressure and high cholesterol.

DON'T SMOKE, unlike 20% of Americans.

TAKE ASPIRIN to reduce your heart attack risk, unlike 20% of American adults.

Little things add up. Don't stop at being healthy or even very healthy. Coming up, advice from doctors on their recommendations to send heart disease packing.

TEST YOUR
HEALTHY-HEART KNOWLEDGE

Small—really small—steps can dramatically slash your risk of America's number one health threat: cardiovascular disease. In fact, the most powerful lifestyle changes you can make to prevent it often seem so tiny that many of us ignore them. Do you? Test your disease-stopping savvy with this quick quiz.

1 HDL cholesterol is super important for heart health. Yours should be:

a. As high as possible

b. As low as possible

c. The same as your spouse's

2 High blood sugar boosts heart disease risk. But doing this can cut your diabetes risk 21%:

a. Exercising one hour a day

b. Eating two extra servings of whole grains a day

c. Giving up carbohydrates

3 You and your heart are carrying around some extra pounds. Does it matter where that excess fat hangs out?

a. Nope. Allover fat's the problem.

b. Yep. Belly fat's the culprit.

c. Yes, that "muffin top" is a concern.

4 If you found out you had slightly elevated blood pressure, you would:

a. Hope it'll go away and try using a little less salt.

b. Ask your doc about medication.

c. Make diet and exercise changes pronto to get it back to normal.

5 If you tweak just one thing in your diet to cut heart-disease risk, it should be:

a. Eliminating gluten

b. Eliminating red meat

c. Cutting out sugary drinks

6 One quirky thing cardiologists do to keep their tickers healthy is:

a. Drinking wine and beer only, never hard liquor

b. De-stressing daily—perhaps by taking a warm, scented bath

c. Getting up at 4 a.m. to run 10 miles

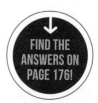

↓

FIND THE ANSWERS ON PAGE 176!

FOLLOW THIS "ROUTINE MAINTENANCE" HEART PLAN

Treat your heart at least as well as you treat your ride. "Just as your car needs regular tune-ups and oil changes to prevent trouble and keep it running at peak, your body needs regular preventive care, too," says Kimberly McMillin, MD, a family practitioner at Baylor Medical Center in Garland, Texas. She and other top docs recommend the following basic but don't-ignore-them checks.

 ## ASK YOUR DOC ABOUT YOUR:

▶ **BLOOD PRESSURE:** Get checked at every doctor visit or at least every one to two years, but more often if you already have prehypertension (a blood pressure reading between 130/80 and 139/89). If you already have high blood pressure, follow your doctor's checkup schedule.

▶ **BLOOD SUGAR:** High levels are a sign of prediabetes or diabetes, and both sharply increase your risk of heart trouble. Get your blood sugar tested at 45, then repeat every three years. Start sooner if you're overweight and have any other diabetes risk factors—family history, inactive lifestyle, high blood pressure, smoking, history of heart disease, a high-risk ethnic background (African American, Latino, Native American, Asian American), a history of diabetes in pregnancy, or giving birth to a baby weighing more than nine pounds.

▶ **CHOLESTEROL AND TRIGLYCERIDE LEVELS:** Starting at age 20, get both checked at least every five years if levels are healthy; more often is optimal. If either or both are already high, follow your doctor's checkup schedule.

SHIELD YOUR TICKER FROM SODA

Most of us grew up with the idea that soda in moderation can be part of a healthy diet. No more. Science now says that just one serving a day can increase your risk of a heart attack.

A can of regular soda packs the equivalent of 14 teaspoons of sugar that, because it's liquid, is absorbed by the body immediately. That's one reason a soda habit lowers HDL, the good cholesterol that deters heart attacks. If my friends or family members still drink regular soda, I tell them to quit.

—JEFF RITTERMAN, MD, CARDIOLOGIST IN RICHMOND, CALIFORNIA

WHY IT WORKS → Unseen and unfelt, sugar from soft drinks and other sources gloms onto proteins in your bloodstream and creates destructive substances called AGEs (short for advanced glycation end products). These encourage wrinkles, stiff joints, heart disease, Alzheimer's, diabetes, kidney problems, bone fractures, and vision loss. And if that's not enough, sugary drinks—soda, sweet tea, fruit punch, and most energy drinks—also raise levels of heart-threatening triglycerides. Smarter sips: unsweetened herbal iced tea or water (plain or carbonated) dressed up with a squeeze of citrus.

MAKE HEART-SMART EATING A NO-BRAINER

A pair of eye-opening studies in 2013 found that one typical restaurant meal contains most of the calories, salt, and fat that an adult should eat in an entire day. Sure, it's possible to find healthy food on menus, but even then today's huge portions and salt-loaded recipes work against you and your heart. Eating at home gives you both a head start.

 WHY IT WORKS → Get ahead of the game with tactics that make home cooking the faster, easier, more affordable choice.

▶ Stock the freezer with quick-cooking chicken breasts or thighs and frozen veggies everyone likes. (Hate frozen peas? Don't buy 'em!)

▶ Keep ready-to-toss bagged salad greens and quick-cooking barley or brown rice on hand for fast side dishes.

▶ Same goes for frozen, unsweetened fruit—puree it into an instant sorbet for dessert with a little sweetener or honey and lemon juice to taste.

Voilà! A dinner your heart and the people you love will adore.

BEAT THE "DIABESITY" HEART THREAT

Experts call it the "diabesity" epidemic, referring to the dual onslaughts of overweight and diabetes threatening the nation. "We urgently need to reverse this. Nearly every piece of your body is damaged by diabetes, starting with your heart and blood vessels—but also including your skin, nervous system, GI tract, kidneys, eyes, and brain," says Francine R. Kaufman, MD, former head of the Center for Diabetes at Children's Hospital, Los Angeles.

The simplest yet often the most powerful way to do this? Change your diet. Don't think about it. Don't procrastinate. Just do it.

CHANGE YOUR DIET.

✔ **DON'T DRINK YOUR CALORIES.** The sugar from juice and soda is so concentrated that it enters your bloodstream immediately and your body has to produce a quick burst of insulin to cope. If it has to do this repeatedly, your odds of weight gain, insulin problems, and diabetes soar. Switch to water or unsweetened iced tea. Make diet soda and drinks with artificial sweeteners an occasional treat.

✔ **GO NATURAL.** Load up on unprocessed goodies (fruit, vegetables, nuts, legumes, lean protein, low-fat dairy) but make a special effort with whole grains. Why? For every extra two servings women eat a day, the risk of type 2 diabetes drops 21%.

✔ **BUY NEW SCALES.** Being just 20 pounds too heavy starts to entice diabetes. The riskiest weight—for your heart, too (see page 172)—is around your middle. Deep abdominal fat pumps out inflammatory chemicals that interfere with your body's ability to absorb blood sugar.

DECIDE TO LIVE TO 100

As people get older, the likelihood for coronary artery disease increases. There is plaque buildup in the body—that's what coronary-artery disease is: your pipes being blocked up with plaque, a sort of sludge. Even teenagers have some plaque.

I find myself being redundant throughout the day. I tell every single patient who comes into the office, whether they're 30 or 80, that they have to do a lot of aerobic exercise, lose weight even if they're just a little heavy, and not smoke. That is the foundation of a healthy cardiovascular approach to long life, regardless of the decade you're in.

—FRED FEUERBACH, MD, ATTENDING CARDIOLOGIST AT NEW YORK-PRESBYTERIAN HOSPITAL AND CARDIOLOGY CONSULTANT AT THE HOSPITAL FOR SPECIAL SURGERY

WHY IT WORKS → Everyone wants to live to 100, but to do that you have to get real. Heart problems are often the result of either cumulative effects (20 years of smoking or not eating right) or genetics. The goal, says Feuerbach, "is that with exercise, cholesterol lowering, and smoking cessation, you can stop plaque buildup and even cause plaque to recede. That's the holy grail."

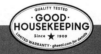

TRY SESAME OIL!

"Sesame oil is a lesser-known source of monounsaturated fats, which are typically touted in olive oil and avocadoes. Swapping sesame for your traditional olive oil gives any sauté or side dish a nutty flavor. For example, try it with snap peas and other heart-healthy ingredients such as garlic and ginger for an extra immune-boost."

—JACLYN LONDON, MS, RD, GOOD HOUSEKEEPING NUTRITION DIRECTOR

TRUST YOUR GUT ABOUT HEART ATTACKS

When girlfriends ask me about heart attack symptoms, I always stress trusting their intuition. Women may not have the crushing chest pain men often do. But almost every female heart attack survivor I've treated has told me that her gut said something was very wrong before she went into cardiac arrest, even if she had no symptoms.

One woman said she felt some arm pain and body aches and had a "funny feeling" about them, but her doctor said the problem was probably muscular. Sure enough, she suffered a massive heart attack, which thankfully she survived.

My point is, if you ever have any symptoms that nag at your intuition—discomfort that's unusual, intense, or just gives you a bad vibe—listen to it, and call 911 right away.

—SUZANNE STEINBAUM, DO, ATTENDING CARDIOLOGIST, DIRECTOR OF WOMEN'S HEART HEALTH AT LENOX HILL HOSPITAL IN NEW YORK CITY, AND AUTHOR OF *DR. SUZANNE STEINBAUM'S HEART BOOK*

 WHY IT WORKS → New research suggests that while the major sign of a heart attack for many women and men *is* crushing chest pain, about one in 10 don't have this symptom. Sneaky warnings that are easy to shrug off or misinterpret can include:

▶ waves of nausea or stomach cramps

▶ shortness of breath without chest pain

▶ sweating, discomfort, or pain in the throat, jaw, neck, or arms, also without chest pain

▶ dizziness and/or bone-deep fatigue—like a weird flu you just can't shake

In one study, men were more likely to have pain down their right arm and shorter episodes of pain. Women were more likely to feel pressure (versus pain) in their chest, be short of breath, or have pain that lasted for 30 minutes.

If you think it's your heart, trust your gut and call 911 immediately. Getting treatment within 90 minutes doubles your chances for survival.

YOUR C-REACTIVE PROTEIN LEVEL. YOUR *WHAT?*

CRP, short for c-reactive protein, is a marker of body-wide inflammation that encourages dangerous blood clots, which can trigger sudden heart attacks and strokes. Even if your cholesterol is normal, men over 50 and women over 60 should ask their doctors to check their CRP levels.

—**NIECA GOLDBERG**, MD, MEDICAL DIRECTOR OF THE JOAN TISCH CENTER FOR WOMEN'S HEALTH AT NYU LANGONE MEDICAL CENTER AND AUTHOR OF *DR. NIECA GOLDBERG'S COMPLETE GUIDE TO WOMEN'S HEALTH*

WHY IT MATTERS → In a study of 17,000 men over 50 and women over 60, those with slightly high levels of CRP cut their heart attack and stroke risk by taking a cholesterol-lowering statin drug—even though they didn't have high cholesterol. That's not the only way to cool inflammation in your body: Losing weight, exercising, and bumping up the fruits and veggies in your diet also help do the trick. Do it. But get a blood test for CRP, too.

HOW TO STOP PREHYPERTENSION

One-third of Americans have prehypertension—a blood pressure reading between 120/80 and 139/80 that means your heart's beginning to work too hard—but there's just not enough awareness about it. It's a window, a chance for you to make aggressive changes that will prevent you from developing deadly high blood pressure down the road. And plenty of research shows that healthy changes make a big difference.

—**SUZANNE STEINBAUM**, DO, ATTENDING CARDIOLOGIST, DIRECTOR OF WOMEN'S HEART HEALTH AT LENOX HILL HOSPITAL IN NEW YORK CITY, AND AUTHOR OF *DR. SUZANNE STEINBAUM'S HEART BOOK*

WHY IT WORKS → "Don't believe the myth that reducing sodium isn't important," Steinbaum says. "Cutting back on salty processed foods and eating a diet packed with produce, lean protein, good fats, and low-fat dairy are proven ways to help. Add a daily walk, and, if you need to, quit smoking, cut back on alcohol, lose weight, and/or manage stress. Do that and you can stop high blood pressure in its tracks."

10-SECOND SOLUTIONS

SHORTEN YOUR WORKDAY
A friend of mine is a high-powered executive who thought she was perfectly healthy—until her doctor discovered a coronary blockage that required a stent. She was shocked and exclaimed to me, "I'm too young for this!" I told her to start leaving the office on time. Studies show that working more than 11 hours a day can raise your odds of heart disease by 67%.

—SHYLA T. VALENTINE, MD, CARDIOLOGIST IN DALLAS

CHECK YOUR WAIST
The larger your waist, the greater your risk of heart trouble—even in people who aren't overweight—found a major study from Harvard and Sweden. Scientists blame the waist-thickening internal fat deep in the abdomen called the omentum. It's linked to big heart threats, including high blood pressure, high blood sugar, high cholesterol, and high triglycerides.

A waist size above 35 inches in women and above 40 in men is a potential risk factor not only for heart disease but also for other conditions, including type 2 diabetes.

—NIECA GOLDBERG, MD, MEDICAL DIRECTOR OF THE JOAN TISCH CENTER FOR WOMEN'S HEALTH AT NYU LANGONE MEDICAL CENTER AND AUTHOR OF *DR. NIECA GOLDBERG'S COMPLETE GUIDE TO WOMEN'S HEALTH*

DON'T TAKE THE PILL AFTER 40

If a friend over 40 mentions that she's on the pill, I'm not shy about telling her to get off it right away. As you get older, you really have to pay attention to hormonal therapies. Birth control pills can lead to blood clots that could cause a heart attack or stroke in your mid-to late 40s.

—**KARLA KURRELMEYER**, MD, CARDIOLOGIST WITH THE HOUSTON METHODIST DEBAKEY HEART AND VASCULAR CENTER IN TEXAS

WHICH BP NUMBER IS MOST IMPORTANT?

I look closely at both blood pressure numbers, but age is a factor. Doctors tend to pay more attention to systolic blood pressure, the top one—which measures pressure *during* a heartbeat—because after 50 it's the most accurate diagnosis of high blood pressure.

But especially in younger people, rising diastolic pressure—the bottom number, which measures pressure *between* heartbeats—can indicate early artery stiffening and a growing risk of heart attacks, strokes and kidney failure. You can often reverse it with exercise and healthy eating.

—**SUZANNE STEINBAUM**, DO, ATTENDING CARDIOLOGIST, DIRECTOR OF WOMEN'S HEART HEALTH AT LENOX HILL HOSPITAL IN NEW YORK CITY, AND AUTHOR OF *DR. SUZANNE STEINBAUM'S HEART BOOK*

WHEN TO WORRY ABOUT CHOLESTEROL

You may think high cholesterol and triglyceride levels are problems your grandfather has. But in my cardiology practice, younger and younger men and women are showing up with high cholesterol. I keep track of mine and tell my patients and the people I love to do the same. At any age, your cholesterol can tell you a lot about the vitality of your heart.

—**SUZANNE STEINBAUM**, DO, ATTENDING CARDIOLOGIST, DIRECTOR OF WOMEN'S HEART HEALTH AT LENOX HILL HOSPITAL IN NEW YORK CITY, AND AUTHOR OF *DR. SUZANNE STEINBAUM'S HEART BOOK*

KNOW YOUR NUMBERS →

"Your total cholesterol should be under 200, but don't focus on the total," Steinbaum says. "Look at your LDL cholesterol. If it's above 130, your risk for heart disease is more than twice as high as it is for someone with normal LDL levels; if it's above 160, your risk triples. Reducing saturated fat, losing weight, and getting exercise will all help. So will cholesterol-lowering statin drugs. It also depends on your other risk factors and if you have had heart disease. The truth is, in those situations, the lower the better, and the goal is less than 100.

"Then look at your HDL cholesterol. It's the good stuff. A man's should be above 40; a woman's, above 50 but aim higher. Getting your HDL over 60 with exercise and healthy eating is highly heart-protective. That's what I want to see in my patients and myself."

· GOOD · HOUSEKEEPING
QUALITY TESTED
Since ★ 1909
LIMITED WARRANTY · ghseal.com for details

"Dip into hummus. Fiber, especially soluble fiber from beans, is linked with improved heart health. And chickpeas are one of the best for giving us a cholesterol-lowering boost: Just ⅓ cup of chickpeas has about 12 grams of fiber—half of your daily value."

—**JACLYN LONDON**, MS, RD, GOOD HOUSEKEEPING NUTRITION DIRECTOR

YOUR "HEART THROBS" ARE SPECIAL

What I always tell my patients is that you are an individual. You need to understand your own unique health profile, which goes beyond cholesterol and blood pressure. We each have our own special "heart throbs"—habits, situations, and genetics that aren't part of a standard cardio test yet deeply influence the health of our heart and arteries.

—SUZANNE STEINBAUM, DO, ATTENDING CARDIOLOGIST, DIRECTOR OF WOMEN'S HEART HEALTH AT LENOX HILL HOSPITAL IN NEW YORK CITY, AND AUTHOR OF *DR. SUZANNE STEINBAUM'S HEART BOOK*

"Heart throbs include your exercise habits, your hormonal status, your sleep quality, and your attitude toward life," Steinbaum says. "For example, we know that people who are physically fit are at lower risk for a heart attack, and people who sit most of the time are at higher risk. Do you get at least 30 minutes of exercise daily and get out of your chair every half hour or so to 'wake up' your muscles, which include your heart?

"Look at your mindset, too. Pessimists face higher heart risks because their stress hormone levels are higher. I work on this myself. Yes, my life is busy. But I do my best not to let things like traffic jams upset me anymore."

Sleep also affects heart health. Heart-disease risk rises if you log less than six or more than 10 hours most nights. And long-term disturbed sleep—due to insomnia, sleep apnea, work/family demands, or other issues—also increases your risk for high blood pressure and heart attacks.

ANSWERS TO
HEALTHY-HEART KNOWLEDGE

1 **A.** Higher is better when it comes to heart-friendly HDLs. These particles help remove heart-threatening LDLs from your body. Target for women: over 50 mg/dL. For men: over 40 mg/dL. *See page 174.*

2 **B.** That's right, adding just two servings of whole grains to your diet can slash your risk for type 2 diabetes significantly. Best way to do it: Swap a refined carb (white bread, white crackers, white rice) for an unrefined one (whole-wheat bread, whole-wheat crackers, brown rice). *See page 168.*

3 **B AND C.** Yep, belly fat— including a "muffin top"—is a heart threat even if your overall weight is in a healthy range. *See page 177.*

4 **C.** One in three Americans has prehypertension (slightly elevated blood pressure). Top docs know that finding out you have this "shadow condition" is a golden opportunity to take lifestyle steps proven to slash risk for progressing to hypertension. *See page 171.*

5 **C.** Cutting out gluten is a must only for people who can't tolerate the protein, which is found in wheat and some other grains. It's true that skipping fatty red meat (bacon, cold cuts, marbled steaks, etc.) can lower your risk for ticker trouble. But health experts say nixing sugar-loaded drinks (soda, shakes, sweet tea, fruit punch, energy drinks, rich coffee concoctions) may be even more powerful, because this "liquid candy" can increase heart-threatening blood fats called triglycerides and trigger other body-chemistry changes that endanger your heart. *See page 168.*

6 **B.** Stress reduction is fast becoming part of the standard get-healthier "prescriptions" written by top docs who are savvy about preventive medicine. In fact, heart experts told us they encourage others and themselves to take time every day to decompress. The bonus? It feels good! *See page 172.*

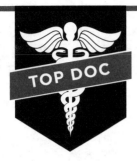

REMEMBER THESE FOUR HEART-SAVING SECRETS

Ready to protect yourself—and the people you love—from America's most threatening disease? These small, doable lifestyle steps MDs recommend taking are *proven* to make the biggest differences. Follow this game plan to put their advice to work in your life:

1 REMEMBER THAT EVERY LITTLE BIT COUNTS. A 10-minute walk, substituting whole-wheat bread for white bread, opting for fruit salad over a jumbo brownie, turning off the TV, and turning in half an hour earlier . . . these steps may seem like no big deal by themselves, but smart little lifestyle changes add up big-time. Ask any doc.

2 MAKE TIME FOR SCREENINGS. Catching the early warning signs for heart disease—rising cholesterol, blood pressure, triglycerides, even rising blood sugar numbers—gives you time to deploy lifestyle changes when they're most effective.

3 CHILL OUT. Schedule feel-good "me time" every day. There's a growing consensus that chronic stress is hard on your blood vessels and your heart.

4 WATCH YOUR WAIST SIZE. Even if the scales say your overall weight is okay, belly fat is a risk factor for high blood pressure, high cholesterol, heart attacks, and strokes. Keep your waist under 35 inches if you're a woman, under 45 if you're a man.

BE A SAVVY HEALTH CONSUMER

TOP DOCS RECOMMEND BEING A SMART HEALTHCARE CONSUMER. When it comes to preventive care, they believe in making great use of the American healthcare system to get the tests and care you need to stay healthy.

In this chapter, top docs open up about what they think their patients should do to navigate the healthcare system. An emergency-room physician reveals how to negotiate the ER. A drug-safety expert shares the extra steps he takes to avoid common—and dangerous—pharmacy errors. A medical records expert has advice on digital healthcare. You'll also find out why you should get a yearly physical and how to be a "top patient."

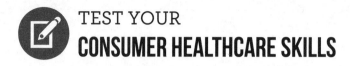

TEST YOUR
CONSUMER HEALTHCARE SKILLS

Smart healthcare consumers play a big role in their own care. That's where top docs have an inside track and plenty to share with the rest of us about everything from sidestepping prescription mistakes and remembering to take pills to avoiding long delays in the waiting room. Can you navigate the healthcare system? Take this quiz, then read the chapter for all the details.

1 The most common prescription drug error made by pharmacists is:

a. Putting the wrong drug in the bottle

b. Giving you someone else's medication

c. Giving you the right drug but the wrong dose

2 For most people, the best check for inherited diseases is:

a. One of those direct-to-consumer gene test kits

b. Creating a family health history

c. A medical lab test of worrisome genes

3 Calling your doctor for results of medical tests is important because:

a. Medical offices are so buried in paperwork that it's wise to keep your own records.

b. One in 14 abnormal test results may not be reported to patients.

c. It's the fastest way to find out if you're okay.

4 The percentage of doctors who've converted from paper files to electronic medical records is:

a. Almost 50%

b. 75%

c. Over 90%

5 You should get a second opinion when:

a. You or a loved one is facing a major, life-threatening disease

b. You have a chronic health problem and wonder if your treatment plan is top-notch

c. Both

d. Neither unless you don't trust your doctor

6 The best way to cut waiting time in your doctor's office is:

a. Fill out all paperwork in advance and mail, fax, or email it back.

b. Get there early, find out how long the wait is, and reschedule if it's forever.

c. Pretend you have an emergency.

FIND THE ANSWERS ON PAGE 194!

GET AN ANNUAL PHYSICAL

I absolutely get a physical every year, along with blood pressure checks, cholesterol tests, a prostate exam, vaccination updates—the whole preventive-medicine routine, including a colonoscopy every five to 10 years. So many of the diseases people wind up with could have been prevented, treated, or cured if they'd been caught early.

The truth is, if you're fairly healthy you can likely get by without much medical intervention for the first 50 years of your life. But after that many systems in your body start hitting a kind of breakdown stage and don't work as well. You have to monitor them to know if something's going wrong so there's time to make healthy changes and get treatments that could save you money, pain, or quite possibly your life.

—**ARTHUR J. MOLLEN**, DO, OSTEOPATHIC FAMILY PHYSICIAN IN SCOTTSDALE, ARIZONA, AND AUTHOR OF SEVERAL BOOKS, INCLUDING *HEALTHONOMICS: THE HANDBOOK FOR BALANCING YOUR PHYSICAL* AND *FINANCIAL CHECKBOOKS*

"Despite recent studies questioning the value of annual physicals, every day I see in my practice why they're so important," says Mollen. "Recently I had a patient who hadn't seen a doctor in a decade. He turned out to have diabetes, high blood pressure, blockages in arteries in his heart, and early stage prostate cancer. We're working on all of those issues, but he was a walking time bomb."

In addition to the physical side of an annual exam, be sure to discuss your emotional health. If your doctor doesn't ask, bring it up, says Mollen. "Here's one good example of why this is important. Depression, which is treatable, may masquerade as fatigue, irritability, rage, even a low sex drive."

AVOID THE NUMBER ONE PHARMACY ERROR

The most common error pharmacists make is accidentally putting someone else's prescription in a bag with your name on it. When I get prescriptions filled for myself or my family, I *never* leave the drugstore without opening the bag and checking the name on the container. Research shows that over half of prescription errors happen this way.

Yet you can totally avoid it with one simple step: Confirm that the right name is on the prescription container itself.

—MICHAEL COHEN, RPH, MS, SCD (HON), DPS (HON), PRESIDENT OF THE INSTITUTE FOR SAFE MEDICATION PRACTICES

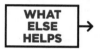

"Even better, when you call in a refill or pick up a prescription, give a second piece of identifying information, like your address or date of birth," says Cohen. "This is especially smart if you have a common name, since a pharmacy may easily have several people on file with names that are the same or very similar to yours." In fact, more pharmacies today now ask not only for your name but also for extra identifying information to avoid exactly this problem, so don't be surprised or reluctant to give it. It protects you as well as them.

Also, know the names of your medications, plus why and how you take them. If any of the information is even a little different from what you expected, tell the pharmacist. Clear up any concerns before using the medication.

DOUBLE-CHECK E-PRESCRIPTIONS

If I'm at a medical appointment and a prescription is sent electronically to my pharmacy, I always ask for a voided copy of my prescription or printout with information about my prescription before I leave. I want to be sure the medication I get at the drugstore is correct—the right name, right strength, right quantity, right directions.

At least 70% of office physicians now prescribe electronically. This is mainly a good thing. It eliminates errors caused by barely legible handwriting. Computers also act as a backup, alerting pharmacists (physicians, too) about possible drug interactions and contraindications that might have been missed.

—MICHAEL COHEN, RPH, MS, SCD (HON), DPS (HON), PRESIDENT OF THE INSTITUTE FOR SAFE MEDICATION PRACTICES

WHY IT WORKS → "With e-prescribing you may not get anything in writing at your doctor's office, and by the time you get to the pharmacy, you may not remember exactly what the drug was or how to take it. Asking for a prescription voucher when your doctor orders an Rx electronically prevents mistakes. The voucher should list the medication, the dose, and the directions," Cohen says. "Compare it with the drug label on the pharmacy container."

GET A CLEAR DIAGNOSIS

There's one thing I always emphasize to family and friends: When something's happening with your health, make sure you get a clear diagnosis before making decisions about tests and treatment. It sounds obvious, but it often isn't, especially when doctors are still running tests or even trying out treatments.

A lot of times docs will say, "Let's do some tests and we'll figure it out." You don't even know what they *think* the problem might be. Probe a bit and try to find out what's in their heads. Knowing this will help you make better decisions about tests and initial treatments. It makes you a more active partner in your care.

—LEANA WEN, MD, EMERGENCY PHYSICIAN AND AUTHOR OF *WHEN DOCTORS DON'T LISTEN: HOW TO AVOID MISDIAGNOSES AND UNNECESSARY TESTS*

WHY IT WORKS → "It helps you avoid overtesting. For example, a doctor may suggest a test with some potentially risky side effects," Wen says. "If it's not going to provide information that will significantly affect your diagnosis or the treatment you're willing to undergo, you may decide the risk isn't worth it." In a nationwide survey, 42% of doctors said they sometimes overtreat patients, including ordering tests that may not be necessary. Extra tests can lead to unneeded treatments, medications, or surgical procedures and cost bundles of money.

TELL YOUR DOCTOR THE WHOLE STORY

My medical training coincided with the "training" I received while caring for my mother when she developed terminal cancer. She was diagnosed when I was in medical school and passed away when I was a resident, so my time with her really informed my education as a physician. One thing I learned was that it's vital to talk to your doctor about your story, not just your symptoms.

What you should tell your doctor is a lot like what you would tell an old friend you haven't seen in a while who asks how you've been. You wouldn't just recite a bunch of facts and figures. You'd tell a story full of depth and nuance and richness. Believe it or not, that same approach is what leads to a good diagnosis 80% of the time.

To be honest, my mother didn't tell her story often enough and didn't let me tell it. I wish I had helped her speak up. The outcome might have been different. She had many misdiagnoses. Initially, her cancer was missed. Then multiple other problems were missed along the way, eventually including the pneumonia that led to her death.

—**LEANA WEN**, MD, EMERGENCY PHYSICIAN AND AUTHOR OF *WHEN DOCTORS DON'T LISTEN: HOW TO AVOID MISDIAGNOSES AND UNNECESSARY TESTS*

 "Speak up the moment you have a question or don't understand something a doctor said, or realize a doctor doesn't understand what you said," Wen says. "Tell your story. Don't let more time and more opportunities for misunderstanding go by."

Cover the same elements reporters do: who, what, when, where, why, and how. Think about your story ahead of time, because you may only have 10 seconds to talk (that's average) before your doc interrupts. Instead of saying, "I have abdominal pain," tell the story: what you ate for dinner, how you felt fine all night but woke up with cramps, then got nauseated, then vomited, then had diarrhea all day. It gives your doctor much more information.

GO METRIC WITH LIQUID MEDS

More and more liquid medications, prescription or not, give dosage information based on the metric system. So it's better to just get used to it.

You should never use household spoons to measure out liquid medicine anyway—they're not accurate. Use whatever measuring device (spoon, cup, oral syringe) comes with the medicine. If it's a dosing cup, put it on a flat surface and check the amount at eye level to be sure your pour is accurate.

Play it safe afterward, too. Replace the cap on the bottle right away. If there are kids around, be sure the cap is child-resistant and locked. Even then, put the bottle out of reach. Wash your measuring tool pronto and store it with the medicine so it's easy to find next time.

—MICHAEL COHEN, RPH, MS, SCD (HON), DPS (HON), PRESIDENT OF THE INSTITUTE FOR SAFE MEDICATION PRACTICES

 → "Studies show that people mismeasure or misunderstand liquid medicine doses as often as 50 to 70% of the time," says Cohen. Measuring out the correct dose can be tricky, especially if it's late or the room is dim. Using the right tools helps you get the safe, correct amount. Turn on a bright light and grab your glasses.

GET THIS CAREGIVING BENEFIT

As a caregiver for my own parents, I found out that it's a lot easier for me to help others than it is to ask others to help me. I'm not unusual. Many caregivers find it hard to accept help when they need it—a condition I playfully call RDD, for Receiving Deficit Disorder.

Surprisingly, caregivers get a benefit few people realize. They enjoy a longevity advantage, according to a recent Johns Hopkins University study of more than 6,000 caregivers and non-caregivers. People who regularly tend to the needs of a family member add nine months to their life expectancy, despite the stress and strain involved. Why? Caregiving can be a loving, deeply meaningful experience.

—YOSAIF AUGUST, AWARD-WINNING HEALTHCARE INNOVATOR AND LIFE COACH, AUTHOR OF *COACHING FOR CAREGIVERS: HOW TO REACH OUT BEFORE YOU BURN OUT*, AND CO-AUTHOR OF *HELP ME TO HEAL*

 Caregivers live longer, researchers say, *if* highly stressful situations can be avoided or managed effectively One of the best ways to do this is to reach out to others who are willing and eager to share the care. If you can't find a way to accept help, you risk burnout from trying to be the sole caregiver. Being able to reach out for help is vital for sustaining the care you're providing, and for your own well-being.

A 12-step program for curing RDD: Strengthen your "reaching out" muscles by asking for help with simple tasks—a little shopping, walking the dog, sitting with your loved one for an hour or two while you run errands. Do this 12 times. Notice how good it feels to lighten your load, and how much your friends and family appreciate the chance to help out.

THE HEALTH SECRETS HIDING IN YOUR FAMILY TREE

A family health history may be the most powerful "genetic test" you'll ever take. Fortunately, I have a large, talkative family on my mother's side. When we get together, everyone loves to share stories about their childhood and talk about problems, including medical ones. As a result, I knew there was no breast cancer on my mother's side.

However, my father's relatives are much more reserved, and I had never asked them about their health. But then one day I got a call from a cousin on my father's side, telling me that his mother had end-stage breast cancer. After we hung up, I called my dad and pressed him for more information about this bad news. That's how I found out that two other aunts on his side of the family had also had breast cancer in the last 10 years, though both were in remission. I got a mammogram.

—**KATHRYN TENG**, MD, FACP, DIRECTOR OF THE CENTER FOR PERSONALIZED HEALTHCARE AT THE CLEVELAND CLINIC, AND ASSISTANT PROFESSOR AT THE CLEVELAND CLINIC LERNER COLLEGE OF MEDICINE, CASE WESTERN UNIVERSITY

 Knowing your family health history helps you and your doctor predict your risk for a variety of conditions—including heart disease, diabetes, and osteoporosis—and set up personalized prevention. It can also help determine whether you're among the small percentage of people who should consider tests for genetic disorders.

SMART WAYS TO NAG YOURSELF

Doctors struggle as much as everyone else when trying to stick with healthy habits, especially since our schedules are so unpredictable. The only way I remember to take my vitamins is to leave a little travel bottle next to my toothbrush. I link yearly medical exams with easy-to-remember events: Back-to-school season signals I'm due for an ob/gyn checkup. My birthday means it's time for a mammogram.

—**MAY HSIEH BLANCHARD**, MD, CHIEF OF GENERAL OBSTETRICS AND GYNECOLOGY, UNIVERSITY OF MARYLAND SCHOOL OF MEDICINE, BALTIMORE

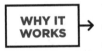 We all need a nudging system to remember to do the things that keep us healthy. Up to 66% of people don't take prescriptions correctly, found a study of 64 million Americans. Need some smart ways to nag yourself?

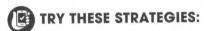 **TRY THESE STRATEGIES:**

▶ **OLD-FASHIONED AND NEW-TECH SYSTEMS:** When volunteers used a pill dispenser that sorts medications into daily compartments, 58% remembered their medicines more often, according to a study by Ohio Northern University. Runners-up included two extremes: text messages—using online reminder apps—and good old-fashioned refrigerator magnets!

▶ **REMINDERS FROM YOUR DOC:** Say yes if your MD asks if you want reminder calls or letters. Researchers say both boost the odds that you'll remember to make appointments for important screenings, like colon cancer tests.

10-SECOND SOLUTIONS

MAKE A GAME PLAN

Never leave a doctor's office without a game plan. Ask when tests will be back and who's going to call whom. One alarming study made it clear how important this is: It found that doctors failed to notify patients of abnormal test results, or record that they'd done so, in one out of 14 cases. Some practices slipped up one out of four times!

—MEHMET OZ, MD, HOST OF THE *DR. OZ SHOW* AND PROFESSOR OF SURGERY, COLUMBIA UNIVERSITY COLLEGE OF PHYSICIANS AND SURGEONS

GET A DOCTOR TO CALL YOU BACK

When you call and ask to talk to your doctor, unless it's an emergency, most receptionists will have doctors call you back. What helps: being specific about when, say receptionists. They suggest saying something like, "I'm only available between two and four. Can the doctor call then?" They'll usually make it happen. Alternatively, ask the receptionist to email the doc on your behalf and copy you; it may produce a quicker response.

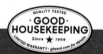

"New health tech is making it easier than ever before to track your medical records. Instead of having everything in tucked-away files or spending hours on the line with your doctor to get your records faxed over, you can have a centralized, digitized personal health history. It will serve as a compilation of all of your health documents, so you can easily collect, organize, and share your data as needed."

—RACHEL ROTHMAN, CHIEF TECHNOLOGIST, GOOD HOUSEKEEPING

HOW TO SEE A DOC FASTER

Front-office receptionists control it all: the calendar, the phones, the email, who gets an appointment when, and who gets seen next. These insider tips from top docs' staffers will help you get faster care when you need it.

1 DO THE PAPERWORK IN ADVANCE. Seeing a new doctor? Ask about doing new-patient paperwork before you go—through email, fax, or electronic medical records. "Most medical offices are switching over to EMRs," says Wendy Winstead, office manager for a Beverly Hills plastic surgeon. "When you call and make an appointment, ask if it's an option; if so, they'll give you a code you can use to log in and file." Ask about faxing paper forms in advance, too.

WHY IT WORKS If the doctor is ahead of schedule, you might get seen right away if your paperwork's complete.

2 MORNINGS ARE MAGIC. If you're trying to reach a physician by phone, call early.

WHY IT WORKS "In the morning, everyone's around to answer the phones. At midday, half the staff is at lunch," says Winstead. Make early morning appointments, too. "The doctor won't be running late due to slow patients ahead of you."

3 WORK THE WAIT LIST. If the first available appointment is months from now, ask for a spot on the waiting list—"then call every day," says Shannon Clark, a receptionist for a physical therapy clinic in New York City.

WHY IT WORKS "When the receptionist realizes you aren't going to stop until your needs are met, you'll likely get the next spot," says Clark.

4 KNOW IF IT'S THAT TIME OF THE YEAR. Find out when your doctor's office is busiest—for example, most offices are extra-busy in November and December because insurance deductibles and some health spending accounts reset on January 1.

WHY IT WORKS Convenient appointments are easier to get and waiting-room times are shorter in slower periods.

WHERE TO GET A SECOND OPINION

I've told many friends and family members to get second opinions for all sorts of medical issues, from a cancer diagnosis to diabetes complications. The result: Many got new information that changed their treatment in important ways.

But what if there isn't a second specialist in your area or you don't live close to a large medical center or you aren't well enough to travel? How do you get a second opinion? *Go online!* Seriously.

Getting a second opinion online from a top medical institution can be an efficient, effective way to get important new information about your condition. Studies of the online second-opinion service at our hospital have found that in 38% of cases, we agree with the recommended treatment. But in 62% of cases, our specialists have recommended minor to major changes. And about 25% of the time, we don't agree with the original diagnosis.

—JONATHAN SCHAFFER, MD, MBA, ORTHOPEDIC SURGEON AT THE CLEVELAND CLINIC AND MANAGING DIRECTOR OF THE CLINIC'S MYCONSULT ONLINE MEDICAL SECOND OPINION SERVICE

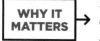

WHY IT MATTERS → More information is always useful. For example, a second opinion may be essential if you're contemplating major surgery or a long-term drug with serious side effects. Ditto if you have a condition that's simply not improving, or you're not convinced your diagnosis is correct, or you simply wonder if there's anything more or different that could be done. Get a second opinion whenever you feel you don't know enough. It doesn't mean you distrust your doctor.

ONLINE HELP FOR OVERWHELMED FAMILIES

When friends are going through a health crisis, it's often hard to find out what's happening or know how to pitch in and help. For overwhelmed families, keeping people posted about an ill person's condition and returning calls and emails is often just one more burden.

Now there's a high-tech but heartwarming solution. In the past few years, several new websites have emerged that I call caresites. They're easy to use and free. The sites allow families to post updates about their loved one, which others can check regularly. Some caresites also have calendars or bulletin boards where families can post things they need help with. This lets friends sign up to assist with what they're good at on days they can do it—without having to bother the family in the process. Caresites also make it easy for you to send messages of love and support.

—**YOSAIF AUGUST**, AWARD-WINNING HEALTHCARE INNOVATOR AND LIFE COACH, AUTHOR OF *COACHING FOR CAREGIVERS: HOW TO REACH OUT BEFORE YOU BURN OUT*, AND CO-AUTHOR OF *HELP ME TO HEAL*

 HOW IT WORKS → Caresites can be as private or as public as you wish. You can limit access only to people you've invited to join, or open it up to anyone who hears about the person in need. Popular sites include www.caringbridge.com, www.lotsahelpinghands.com, and www.carepages.com. "I've participated in several caresites," August adds. "Some are small and intimate. Others have grown to include thousands of people around the world who have created prayer circles and found other ways of showing support."

ANSWERS TO
CONSUMER HEALTHCARE SKILLS

1 **B.** Over half of all prescription drug errors happen when someone else's drug is put in your bag. So *always* open the bag and check the container label before leaving the pharmacy. Be sure it has the right name and the right drug at the correct dose. *See page 182.*

2 **B.** Knowing your family health history can help you and your doctor predict your risk for a wide variety of conditions, including heart disease, diabetes, osteoporosis, and some cancers—and devise a plan to protect you against them. *See page 188.*

3 **B.** In one study, troubling medical test results that needed follow-up care weren't reported to patients in as many as one in 14 cases. That's one good reason to keep track of the tests you've had—and to know when to expect the results, so you can call in if your doctor's office doesn't contact you. *See page 190.*

4 **C.** More than 90% of doctors now use electronic medical records rather than paper files—though during the transition you may see both in use. That may be one reason just 29% of Americans said their docs were moving to digital record keeping in 2013. Finding out what your doctor is doing can make you a more active partner in your care if the system gives you access to your files from home, as some do. *See page 190.*

5 **C.** Second opinions aren't just for enormous, life-threatening health crises. Consulting with an additional specialist can give you peace of mind and maybe a new treatment approach if you're dealing with a chronic health condition such as diabetes, arthritis, heart disease, or asthma. If you can't get to a large medical center for a consultation, consider one of the online second-opinion services run by some of America's leading hospitals. *See page 192.*

6 **A.** Doctors' receptionists say taking care of paperwork ahead of time can speed up the office wait time—if you're ready to be seen the moment you arrive, they may be able to squeeze you in. *See page 191.*

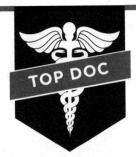

TOP DOC

DEAL WITH THE HEALTHCARE SYSTEM LIKE A PRO

Follow the same strategies top docs use for themselves and their families.

1 **DOUBLE CHECK WHEN BUYING AND TAKING MEDICATIONS.** Picking up a prescription? *Open the bag and check the label at the pharmacy.* Doc filling out an electronic prescription? *Get a copy for yourself.* Doling out liquid medicines in the middle of the night? *Turn on the lights, grab your glasses, and take your time.*

2 **DON'T TRUST YOUR MEMORY!** Up to two out of three of us don't take prescription medications as directed and as a result don't get their full benefit. Even docs use reminder systems. Find one that works for you—a pill dispenser, apps that send you pill-time alerts, a refrigerator magnet that says "take your meds," electronic pill-bottle caps that blink or beep. Your health is worth it.

3 **BE HONEST WITH YOURSELF.** Understand your health risks. Do you have a family health history of early stroke, arthritis, or another condition? What about your own past? Did or do you have a habit (or two) that increases your odds for future health trouble? Get real by knowing where you stand. Then use your resources to make smart changes. Take advantage of health tests, gym memberships, weight-loss programs, and nutrition counseling covered by your insurance, for example. And talk with your doc about other strategies that would help.

4 **BE HONEST WITH DOCS.** Whether you're in the emergency room, getting a routine exam, or meeting with a specialist, tell them everything. Don't ramble, but do describe what's happened and why you're worried. Be honest about less-than-stellar health habits—smoking, alcohol use, eating and exercise habits, drug use. Docs aren't there to scold. They need the whole story in order to give you great care.

5 **HAVE AN ANNUAL WELLNESS VISIT.** Sure, your doc could probably shoehorn a cholesterol or blood sugar test into that 15-minute flu shot visit. But that's not smart preventive health. Health insurance usually covers a routine wellness exam—and for women, an annual or biannual pelvic exam, mammogram, and Pap test. Physicians consider an annual checkup the best way to spot potential problems early. Go for it.

MENTAL HEALTH & HAPPINESS

IN THIS CHAPTER, YOU'LL DISCOVER INGENIOUS WAYS TOP HEALTH practitioners recommend to boost your happiness and bolster your brain health to support clear thinking and a razor-sharp memory.

How do physicians recommend keeping your brain sharp and attitude optimistic?

WORK-LIFE BALANCE: How can you balance a tsunami of on-the-job stress and prevent burnout?

FAITH OR SPIRITUALITY: Spiritual health can be a powerful way to see your glass as half full.

A STRONG MARRIAGE: Only 55% of Americans who've walked down the aisle are in their first marriage. How can you make your relationships last and keep them fresh?

A HAPPY FAMILY: 27% of Americans live alone, which has been shown to negatively impact physical health.

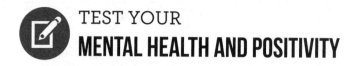

TEST YOUR
MENTAL HEALTH AND POSITIVITY

Feel like you need a brain tune-up? You're not alone. One in eight baby boomers confesses to troubling memory lapses. (Where *are* those car keys?) And the average American today is less happy than the average American was back in the 1950s. Think you're an exception? Test your life skills here, then start learning what docs recommend to keep your brain sharp and your mood sunny.

1 Trading back massages with your spouse or partner can do this:

a. Reduce any conflict between you

b. Decrease blood pressure and increase oxytocin, the "contentment" hormone

c. Set you both up for extra-good sex and sleep

2 To grow new brain cells and stimulate new connections between them:

a. Get regular exercise

b. Eat plenty of lean protein

c. Take special "brain food" dietary supplements

3 **True or false:** Eating lots of superfoods (like blueberries and salmon) could reduce your risk for dementia or delay its development.

4 Belonging to a close-knit group—a book club, faith community, choir, volunteer team, or simply good friends you see often—has this surprising health benefit:

a. A healthier weight

b. A longer life

c. A lower risk of heart disease

5 When you're driving, switching from news radio to a station that plays your favorite songs could:

a. Make you happier

b. Reduce your stress and blood pressure levels

c. Keep you from grinding your teeth

6 Intentionally focusing on small, unimportant details in the world around you can:

a. Enhance spatial awareness

b. Build brainpower and sharpen your memory

c. Make you feel more connected to people and places

FIND THE ANSWERS ON PAGE 216!

HUG A LOT. IT'S REAL MEDICINE

Nothing rejuvenates me faster than spending time with the people I love most in the world. My wife and I make a point of hugging every day long enough to really sink into it.

Besides, research shows that hugging reduces physical and emotional stress that can harm your health and zap your energy. Many studies prove that people with loving relationships and good social connections are healthier. Hugging and touch are good medicine.

One example: When 34 young married couples massaged each other's necks, shoulders and foreheads for half an hour three times a week, researchers at Brigham Young University found that the supportive, caring touch reduced the couples' stress hormones, lowered their blood pressure, and increased their levels of oxytocin, the "cuddle hormone," which promotes feelings of contentment.

—**DAVID L. KATZ**, MD, MPH, FACPM, FACP, FOUNDING DIRECTOR OF YALE UNIVERSITY'S PREVENTION RESEARCH CENTER, PRESIDENT OF THE AMERICAN COLLEGE OF LIFESTYLE MEDICINE, AND AUTHOR OF *DISEASE-PROOF: THE REMARKABLE TRUTH ABOUT WHAT MAKES US WELL*

Touch changes your body chemistry for the better. It activates pressure receptors under the skin called Pacinian corpuscles, which have a direct line to nerves deep in your brain that affect heart rate and blood pressure. Pleasant, friendly touch also lights up your orbitofrontal cortex, a brain area involved with pleasure. That's the science. The feeling? A sense of deep-down well-being. Connecting regularly with loved ones is good for mind, body, and soul.

RECHARGE WITH MUSIC

I listen to music, usually classical or rock, on the way home from work to unwind and get into family mode. I think transition time is really important, especially if you're super busy.

I have a 30-minute commute. My children are grown now, but when they were young, listening to music in the car helped me transition out of my role as Dr. Phelan and into my role as Mrs. Evans, soccer mom and Girl Scout leader.

Now, using this time to relax allows me to switch roles, from being a physician caring for others to being a woman caring for my husband and myself. I enjoy some classical music, like the *Grand Canyon Suite*, *Peter and the Wolf*, and the *Carnival of the Animals*. Otherwise, it's rock and country.

—SHARON PHELAN, MD, FACOG, PROFESSOR OF OBSTETRICS AND GYNECOLOGY AT THE UNIVERSITY OF NEW MEXICO SCHOOL OF MEDICINE, ALBUQUERQUE

 DON'T UNDERESTIMATE THE MIND-BODY BENEFITS OF MUSIC.

▶ Hearing a favorite song stimulates the same brain regions that light up when you're hugged (see above) or eat a favorite food, whether it's caviar or chocolate.

▶ A daily dose of music reduces high blood pressure by four points (on par with cutting back on salt or exercising more), according to one Italian study.

▶ Relaxing with music lowers stress hormones better than chilling out in silence, say Swedish researchers.

▶ And it eases anxiety as effectively as massage, found a Seattle study.

The only secret? Listening to music *you* love—that's when its powers emerge. As long as you like what you're hearing, everything works, from Kenny Rogers and Frank Sinatra to Bach and Celtic folk songs.

TAP INTO THE FIDO EFFECT

I have two little rescue dogs, Lili and Luci. I make a point of spending time with them in the evening, for their benefit and my own. I bought a laptop specifically for this reason, so even if I need to work at night I can still sit on the couch with a dog on either side. I love it when one of them rests her head on my arm and falls asleep! Lots of research shows that the human-animal bond has real health benefits:

THE POWER OF PETS

✔ Pet owners get more exercise than people without pets.

✔ People confide in their pets and nurture them.

✔ Animals can be great healers—a pet can help lower your blood pressure and cholesterol level.

Pets can be incredibly attuned to people. They develop a sense of you that can improve the quality of your life and even affect how long you live.

—ALAN BECK, SCD, DIRECTOR OF THE CENTER OF THE HUMAN-ANIMAL BOND AT PURDUE UNIVERSITY AND CO-AUTHOR OF *BETWEEN PETS AND PEOPLE: THE IMPORTANCE OF ANIMAL COMPANIONSHIP*

 Many studies point to a connection between overall well-being and spending time with a loved animal. Pet owners have more self-esteem and are less lonely and fearful than petless people, according to a Miami University study—where researchers also found, not surprisingly, that active dogs also reduce your risk of becoming overweight!

REPEAT AFTER ME: "THIS WILL BE A GREAT DAY"

In the first minutes of the morning, when I wake up and get out of bed, I repeat a positive affirmation to myself, like "Wow, this is going to be a terrific day!" There's enough research to show that if you just tell yourself you're going to have a great, healthy day, you'll have a much more positive, productive outlook, even if you don't believe it!

I started doing this years ago after staying at a place with a healthy, outdoors lifestyle. Every morning, my wake-up call included this: "Good morning, today's going to be a great day!" It would get me thinking, "This really *is* going to be a great day." It shows just how powerful your mind is at instilling behavior and attitude adjustments.

That original "great day" affirmation is still one of my morning favorites. But it's good to change things up. Others I use include "I love being healthy and productive," "I feel happy and energized," "I can't wait to exercise because I always feel so good afterward," and "I am such a morning person! I love this time of day"—though I realize that might not work for everyone!

—DAWN JACKSON BLATNER, RDN, CSSD, AUTHOR OF *THE SUPERFOOD SWAP*

"Even if you're wiped out, positive affirmations help you rally and you get more good stuff done as a result," Blatner says. "No matter what obstacles you face in the morning, remember that it's easy to focus on negative stuff, but positivity is what really motivates us."

TAKE CHARGE OF YOUR DEBT— IT'S GOOD FOR YOUR HEALTH

The economic turmoil of the past few years has been incredible, and it showed in my patients. I saw financial worries translate into insomnia, high blood pressure, headaches, stomach pain, acid reflux, smoking, overeating, and overdoing alcohol. New medical advice I now give to others—and myself—is simple: Do all you can to reduce debt.

I have patients at every income level who live paycheck to paycheck and spend a lot of their income on payments for high-interest credit cards and other loans. The better you get at scaling back and living within your means, the lower your financial stress will be. Even if you don't make a lot of money, save small amounts. Pack your lunch. Skip fancy coffee drinks. If you still smoke, join a free online program and quit—you'll save a bundle on cigarettes, not to mention its social costs and health risks.

Just don't skip on essential prescriptions or needed healthcare when money is tight. It will backfire in risks and expenses. Explain your situation to your doctor—you're not the first. Then work out a payment plan with the office manager, ask about medication samples, switch to less-expensive generic drugs if you haven't yet, and see if your doc can help you qualify for low-cost drug programs run by pharmaceutical companies.

—ARTHUR J. MOLLEN, DO, OSTEOPATHIC FAMILY PHYSICIAN IN SCOTTSDALE, ARIZONA, AND AUTHOR OF SEVERAL BOOKS, INCLUDING *HEALTHONOMICS: THE HANDBOOK FOR BALANCING YOUR PHYSICAL* AND *FINANCIAL CHECKBOOKS*

 WHY IT WORKS → "Even mini savings add up over time. And every little bit of debt you pay off reduces those killer interest charges and incredible stress levels," says Mollen.

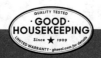

THREE FOODS TO EAT WHEN YOU'RE STRESSED

1. **CHOCOLATE.** The cocoa in chocolate has been linked to boosting levels of the neurotransmitter serotonin, a feel-good chemical in the brain that helps you de-stress *and* feel happier. Since having a small serving of chocolate daily has been linked with improving symptoms of depression and lowering body mass index, you've got a whole lot to feel *lighter* about!

2. **BANANAS WITH ALMOND BUTTER.** The B vitamins in bananas, like folate and vitamin B6, help to serve as cofactors in the production of serotonin, which can help improve mood and reduce anxiety. For an extra stress-busting boost, try topping bananas with almond, peanut, or cashew butter. Since nuts and nut butters are rich in magnesium and zinc, adding them to your meals and snacks can also aid in alleviating both physical *and* emotional stress.

3. **SALMON WITH SPINACH AND TOASTED PINE NUTS.** Aim to eat this omega-3-packed fish (or any other oceanic counterpart!) at *least* twice a week to help de-stress. The omega-3s found in fatty fish, like tuna and salmon, have been linked to decreasing risk of depression and reducing symptoms of anxiety. The bonus: iron- and magnesium-packed spinach and pine nuts can help improve oxygen flow to your cells and aid in muscle contraction—a perfect trio that can help you feel more energized when you're in a stress-slump.

—**JACLYN LONDON**, MS, RD, GOOD HOUSEKEEPING NUTRITION DIRECTOR

TRY PET THERAPY WITHOUT A PET

You can get many of the benefits of pet ownership without owning one. As an adult, I didn't have a dog for quite a while. But I spent time watching animals. I always have. Finding ways to feel tuned in with nature—going to the zoo or the beach, watching fish in an aquarium or birds at a feeder—has proven health benefits.

The benefits of petless pet therapy go further. In research with Nancy Edwards, PhD, RN, we placed aquariums in the dining rooms of nursing homes for people with Alzheimer's—just the presence of the fish was soothing. People who had become less and less interested in food ate 25% more at meals and gained needed weight.

And when we set up fish tanks in dentists' offices, people who saw the swimming fish before their dental treatment felt less pain and had lower blood pressure during their procedures. Dentists, take note!

—**ALAN BECK**, SCD, DIRECTOR OF THE CENTER OF THE HUMAN-ANIMAL BOND AT PURDUE UNIVERSITY AND CO-AUTHOR OF *BETWEEN PETS AND PEOPLE: THE IMPORTANCE OF ANIMAL COMPANIONSHIP*

 WHY IT WORKS → "Studies show that people who connect with the natural world have less depression and anxiety, recover faster from surgery, and may have stronger immunity and even better blood sugar control," points out Beck. "That's good news for anyone who loves animals but doesn't live in a situation where a pet is possible."

SING!

Singing can be very therapeutic. Songs often unlock strong, surprising feelings, memories, and associations. There are songs I play and sing when certain feelings are blocked and I need to release them.

If you think you can't sing, "toning" is a perfect alternative and may even overcome that belief. Take a deep breath and release it with a groan or yawning sound. Keep repeating this until you find a tone that feels comfortable. Let the sound take you wherever it wants to go. Don't try to control it. Ride on the breath. Experiment. Explore. Enjoy.

Whether you sing or tone, you have to breathe deeply to sustain the notes you create. This produces vibrations that nurture the body and massage your insides. Your voice helps you connect to your body and express your emotions. If you're comfortable singing with others around, it also helps you connect to them.

Pay attention to your inner DJ. Is it playing a song? Think about the words and the music you hear in your head. What are they telling you? Your unconscious is probably sending you a message, the way dreams sometimes do.

—**DIANE AUSTIN**, DA, ACMT, LCAT, DIRECTOR OF THE MUSIC PSYCHOTHERAPY CENTER IN NEW YORK CITY AND ADJUNCT PROFESSOR OF MUSIC THERAPY AT NEW YORK UNIVERSITY

WHY IT WORKS → Science has uncovered plenty of health benefits for people who sing, whether you do it alone in the shower, with your family, in a choir, or even with a vocal coach. Singing lowers your levels of the stress hormone cortisol. It also boosts an infection-fighting compound called immunoglobulin A, eases anxiety, and may lift depression a bit.

STUCK? THINK A-B-C-D-E

When you hit a pothole or dead-end as you pursue your goals and propel yourself forward in life, try using the A-B-C-D-E approach—acceptance, bravery, compassion, drive, energy.

A: ACCEPT an obstacle for what it is rather than resisting it. Remember the mandate of biology—every cell is doing the best it can with the resources at hand. Rumination on a stumbling block can deepen the hole you sense you are in. (*I messed up by overeating. I'm hopeless because I missed my workout.*)

B: BRAVELY welcome obstacles and challenges. Hello, look who is here. Be courageous and get curious about new perspectives. Harvest the gift of learning from slip-ups and move forward.

C: FEEL A LITTLE COMPASSION for yourself when your goals are thwarted. Negative emotions such as impatience, anger, worry, sadness, and anxiety are like crying infants: They yearn to be held and loved for a bit. Cross your hands over your heart for a moment of comforting.

D: DRIVE TOWARD THE LARGER PURPOSE you're pursuing. When you're in touch with your truest purposes (*I want to be a great role model for my kids. I want to be resilient so I can handle what's ahead*) meaning and motivation energize your brain's function and energize you to better adapt to the unexpected.

E: FEEL THE ENERGY you get from new insights and new ways to move ahead. You are getting better. Setbacks are really forward leaps in disguise. How energizing is that!

—**MARGARET MOORE**, MBA, CO-FOUNDER AND CO-DIRECTOR OF THE INSTITUTE OF COACHING AT MCLEAN HOSPITAL IN BELMONT, MASSACHUSETTS; CEO OF WELLCOACHES CORPORATION; AND CO-AUTHOR OF *ORGANIZE YOUR MIND, ORGANIZE YOUR LIFE* AND *ORGANIZE YOUR EMOTIONS, OPTIMIZE YOUR LIFE*

WHY IT WORKS → The A-B-C-D-E strategy can help you get past a wide variety of challenges that could otherwise derail you from your goals, whether they're keeping your weight stable, staying focused on a big project, sleeping better, listening more attentively to your friends/family—or all of the above and more.

FOUR WAYS TO FIX MEMORY OVERLOAD

You lost your car in a vast mall parking lot, forgot to pick up your kid after soccer practice, ditzed on the name of that new neighbor. Are you losing your mind? Probably not. Stress, too many distractions, too much multitasking, not enough sleep—all can get in the way of remembering both important and incidental things.

Smart small changes can help get your memory back in shape. Here's how experts in four different disciplines recommend attacking memory lapses caused by overload.

1 THE PSYCHOLOGIST

REPEAT YOURSELF. Locking the door, taking your vitamins, unplugging the iron . . . there's a reason they're called mindless tasks. To help get a routine activity lodged in your brain, say it out loud as you do it ("I'm popping my multi").

WHY IT WORKS The same trick—repeating aloud "I'm getting the scissors"—fends off distraction as you head to the kitchen for them. Memory experts also advise repeating a person's name as you're introduced ("Hi, Alice") and when you finish your conversation ("Nice talking with you, Alice"), but if that feels forced, just repeat the name to yourself as you walk away recommends Cynthia Green, PhD, president of Total Brain Health, a company that provides memory fitness training.

2 THE MEMORY RESEARCHER

DOODLE. Zoning out during a meeting? Sketch something on your notepad. People who color in shapes while listening to someone speak are 29% more likely to recall the information they hear than non-doodlers, according to a report in *Applied Cognitive Psychology*.

WHY IT WORKS "Doodling stops you from daydreaming. You can still listen while doing it, whereas daydreaming reduces your attention to what's being said," says Jackie Andrade, PhD, professor of psychology at Plymouth University, Plymouth, England.

3 THE EXERCISE EXPERT
TAKE A STROLL BEFORE YOUR NEXT BIG PRESENTATION. A 20- to 30-minute power walk is enough to significantly improve your brainpower for about an hour. In studies, people do better on difficult attention tests 30 minutes after doing cardio.

WHY IT WORKS According to Charles Hillman, PhD, professor of kinesiology at the University of Illinois, Aerobic exercise has beneficial effects on both brain structure and brain function that underlie our ability to perform high-level functions (i.e., attention, memory). That's likely to improve your ability to learn new things.

4 THE MINDFULNESS ADVOCATE
TAKE A SECOND LOOK. When you walk a familiar route, look up and down both sides of the street. Notice businesses or homes you've never noticed before and try to notice new things about those you think you already know well.

WHY IT WORKS Even if you'll never need the information, observing and recalling new details gets you off autopilot, and that sharpens your memory. "Not knowing keeps you attentive," says Ellen Langer, PhD, professor of psychology at Harvard University who has written extensively about mindfulness.

FIVE WAYS TO BUILD A SHARPER BRAIN AT ANY AGE

"We used to think that with age, brain cells shriveled up, died and that was that," says Paul Laurienti, MD, PhD, a brain researcher at Wake Forest University School of Medicine. "Now we know that even older brains can grow new, stronger connections."

Brain experts are discovering that making small, everyday changes—like eating a more Mediterranean diet and taking a few brisk walks each week—can build brain volume and create healthy new connections between brain cells. A bigger, better-connected brain reduces your risk for dementia, improves memory, and sharpens fuzzy thinking. Five key changes top brain docs want you to make:

1 **TAKE A WALK.** Yes, you've probably read that 57 times in this book, but only because that's how good walking is for every part of you, including your gray matter.

WHY IT WORKS When you're active, your brain pumps out neurotrophins, compounds that act like fertilizer for new brain cells and connections. Also, a study of older adults found that the brain's hippocampus—an area responsible for memories—is larger in people who are physically active, says Art Kramer, PhD, of the University of Illinois, co-author of the study. Even if you've been sedentary most of your life, getting fitter now will increase the volume of your brain. Get out and walk for an hour a day, even just a few days a week.

2 **PLAY MIND GAMES.** Doing something mentally challenging, like memorizing the constellations or learning basic Chinese, creates fresh brain connections.

3 **DON'T FORGET TO EXERCISE.** Regular exercise is considered to be the single most effective lifestyle change you can make to slow progression of dementia. Even 20 minutes of fast walking three times per week is enough to make a big difference.

WHY IT WORKS You can actually generate new cells in the hippocampus, and those new cells are important for creating new memories. They may protect against memory loss and dementia later in life, according to Peter J. Snyder, PhD, professor of neurology at the Warren Alpert School of Medicine, Brown University.

4 **SLEEP ON IT.** Different areas of your brain collaborate to consolidate and store memories—for instance, connecting a face, a name, and where you met.

WHY IT WORKS Sleep helps knit all those memories together, says Gary Richardson, MD, senior research scientist at the Sleep Disorders Center at Henry Ford Hospital in Detroit. No wonder skimping on your ZZZs is linked with poorer memory later in life.

5 **FEED YOUR LITTLE GRAY CELLS.** Yes, there is such a thing as brain food. Various studies suggest that your neurons love specific nutrients. Here's what and why they work.

▶ **BEANS AND GREENS.** They're rich in folic acid, a B vitamin that improves memory and information-processing speed, according to research on more than 800 adults.

▶ **BERRIES.** Packed with cell-protecting flavonoids, two or more ½ cup servings a week delayed the onset of Alzheimer's by 2.5 years in one study.

▶ **SALMON, SARDINES, MACKEREL, AND OTHER COLD-WATER FISH.** People who have higher blood levels of the DHA form of omega-3s, found in cold-water fish, cut their dementia risk by 47%, compared to those with the lowest levels, according to a study of more than 800 older women and men. Aim for three fish servings a week, or take a daily DHA omega-3 supplement (see page 53).

10-SECOND SOLUTIONS

THINK IN CHUNKS

Because your brain can process only so much information at a time, try chunking bits together. By repeating a phone number as "38, 27" instead of "3, 8, 2, 7," you only have to remember two numbers, not four. If you need to buy ground beef, milk, lettuce, cereal, and buns, think "dinner" (burgers, buns, lettuce) and "breakfast" (cereal and milk).

—**GARY SMALL**, MD, DIRECTOR OF THE UCLA LONGEVITY CENTER

YOU'VE GOTTA HAVE FRIENDS

One lesson I've learned from years of studying people who are at least 100 years old—and still healthy—is the importance of friends and family. Meaningful social connections are definitely a key to longevity. One personal result is that I've made an effort to spend even more time with my own friends and family.

—**BRADLEY WILLCOX**, MD, MS, CO-PRINCIPAL INVESTIGATOR OF THE OKINAWA CENTENARIAN STUDY AND CO-AUTHOR OF *THE OKINAWA DIET PLAN: GET LEANER, LIVE LONGER, AND NEVER FEEL HUNGRY*

GET OFF LIFE'S HAMSTER WHEEL

It's easy to slide into a new day feeling trapped by an endless to-do list. Soon your energy is dwindling, your drive waning, and all you see ahead is nonstop, uninspiring tasks. So look for something creative to do early in the day—something new, something exciting, something that makes you feel alive, not just stuck on life's hamster wheel.

You want to aim for the brain state often described as "flow" or "streaming." It's a creative zone in which you allow yourself to be swept up and fully absorbed in an activity that combines your strengths with just the right dose of challenge—enough to be inspiring but not so much that it makes you anxious.

—**MARGARET MOORE**, MBA, CO-FOUNDER AND CO-DIRECTOR OF THE INSTITUTE OF COACHING AT MCLEAN HOSPITAL IN BELMONT, MASSACHUSETTS; CEO OF WELLCOACHES CORPORATION; AND CO-AUTHOR OF *ORGANIZE YOUR MIND, ORGANIZE YOUR LIFE* AND *ORGANIZE YOUR EMOTIONS, OPTIMIZE YOUR LIFE*

 WHY IT WORKS → "When you're in 'flow,' you don't think about yourself and you aren't distracted or twitchy. You're intensely focused," Moore says. "You feel fully alive, awake, energized, and present. You take risks. You lose your sense of time, may not notice hunger or thirst, and feel uplifted when the experience ends."

Yet in one survey, only 23% of people said they experienced flow often and 40% said they rarely or never enjoyed the feeling. That may be because most of us actually have our flow experiences at work, but we're too distracted to enjoy them fully. Turn off your devices, close your door, put the to-do list out of sight, and feel the flow!

GO ON A "SAVORING ADVENTURE"

This is something my mother taught me as a child—to savor the good times. Now, it's the focus of my research. Studies show that savoring life's good moments increases happiness.

Late in my mother's life, we drove into a forest near her home and sat together in silence, sharing the things we noticed with a laugh or a wink. The colors, the rainbow light in the clouds, the wind rippling the creek. It was intensely beautiful and precious.

Your own savoring adventure can be anything you enjoy—a walk in the woods; cooking or eating a meal you love; an amazing trip to the city, mountains, or seaside. Before you go, really anticipate how wonderful it will be. During the experience, focus on all the sensations and feelings you're having. Use all five senses and don't censor anything.

Express your emotions to whomever you're with. If you're alone, write them down and tell someone about it later. Reminiscing is an important part of savoring life's good moment.

—FRED B. BRYANT, PHD, PROFESSOR OF PSYCHOLOGY AT LOYOLA UNIVERSITY CHICAGO AND AUTHOR OF *SAVORING: A NEW MODEL OF POSITIVE EXPERIENCE*

WHY IT WORKS → Some of the science behind savoring: Bryant had 101 volunteers keep diaries for a month about pleasant experiences and how they reacted to them. Savorers immersed themselves in the good moments, expressed their wonder (some laughed or even shouted), and recounted them to others later. Squelchers told themselves they didn't deserve a good time, looked for imperfections, and focused on how it would all be over soon. Not surprisingly, the savorers experienced more pleasure. Be like them.

HOW GOOD IS YOUR MEMORY?

What color hair did the barista who made your latte this morning have? Was the first man you saw today wearing a blue tie, red tie, or no tie? Playing this game with yourself helps train your brain to focus and retain, strengthening your memory, says Gary Small, MD, UCLA professor of psychiatry and aging, director of the UCLA Longevity Center, and co-author of *2 Weeks to a Younger Brain.* Test your recall with this quiz from Small, then use the research-based advice in this section to improve your memory today and build a better, younger brain for the future.

INSTRUCTIONS Set a timer for two minutes and study the list of 10 words below. When the bell rings, put the list aside, set the timer for 20 minutes, and do something else for a bit—check email, pay bills, read a magazine. When the bell rings again, write down as many words as you can recall (in any order).

Violin	**Cradle**
Balloon	**Mast**
Stereo	**Lizard**
Building	**Teacher**
Strawberry	**Oven**

 ## WHAT THE NUMBER OF WORDS YOU REMEMBERED MEANS

▶ **8 OR MORE:** You're a memory superstar. Make sure you follow the brain-building strategies in this section so you'll keep your title.

▶ **5 TO 7:** This is typical for a middle-aged person. Adopting some of the brain-boosting tricks on these pages will boost your score, and your memory.

▶ **4 OR FEWER:** Your memory bank needs an upgrade. Actively use many of the tips in this chapter for better short-term memory recall as well as brain-building strategies.

ANSWERS TO
MENTAL HEALTH AND POSITIVITY

1 | **B.** When married couples get physically close—massaging each other's necks, shoulders, and foreheads for half an hour three times a week—their stress hormones dropped. So did their blood pressure, while levels of the contentment hormone oxytocin rose. A great reason to truly stay in touch with your partner. *See page 199.*

2 | **A.** Getting regular exercise does your brain good. Plenty of research proves that exercise encourages the growth of new brain cells and new connections between them. One study found that the hippocampus, a brain area responsible for forming memories, is bigger in regular exercisers than in couch potatoes. *See page 210.*

3 | **TRUE.** Having just two small servings of berries weekly could delay the development of Alzheimer's disease by 2.5 years—due, perhaps, to phytochemicals that rev up the body's cell-protecting anti-oxidant defenses. Regularly eating cold-water fish like salmon (mackerel, trout) that are packed with omega-3 fatty acids could reduce dementia risk by as much as 47%. *See page 210.*

4 | **B.** Close friends help you live longer. That's one conclusion of researchers who've spent years studying some of the world's longest-living people: healthy 100-year-olds in Okinawa, Japan. You may get similar benefits from building and maintaining valuable friendships. *See page 212.*

5 | **C.** The sound of your favorite songs does more than keep your toes tapping. Research shows that hearing music you love lights up the same brain regions as eating chocolate. It's also as relaxing as a massage, one study found, and can lower tension, anxiety, and blood pressure. No wonder they call it "music therapy"! *See page 200.*

6 | **B.** Intentionally noticing more details around you—in your home, on your commute, at the store—trains you to remember more, brain-health experts say. It's just one way to increase brainpower as you go about your day. Others include walking, repeating little things out loud, and even doodling during a presentation. *See page 208.*

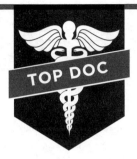

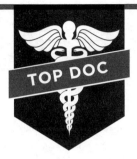TOP DOC

REMEMBER THESE FIVE STRATEGIES FOR STAYING SMART AND UPBEAT

A sharper brain. A brighter, lighter mood. Just being able to find your phone in the morning. They're all great mental health and fitness goals. In this chapter, top docs shared more than two dozen strategies for doing this. Here, they're condensed into this easy-to-follow, five-step action plan:

1 MAKE TIME FOR TOUCH. A cuddle with your spouse or partner. A hug from your best friend. Even petting your dog or cat—or a neighbor's. There's good and growing evidence that human touch increases happiness and changes your body chemistry for the healthier by reducing stress hormones and blood pressure.

2 EXERCISE TODAY. REPEAT TOMORROW. There's a reason physical activity tops the list of top docs' "get happy, stay sharp" advice. Science shows movement can reduce depression, increase energy, and actually stimulate the growth of new brain cells and new links between them. A 30-minute daily walk could make you mentally younger, smarter, and more joyful.

3 TRAIN YOUR BRAIN. There's plenty of evidence that real mental challenges—learning a new language, playing well-designed brain games on your computer, memorizing the constellations—can increase aspects of brain sharpness and memory.

4 LIVE A FULL LIFE. Make time for friends, music, and deep enjoyment of places and experiences you really love. You'll reduce your stress—itself a proven way to reduce brain wear and tear—and increase your happiness and possibly your life span.

5 FEED YOUR BRAIN. Say yes to good fats—the omega-3s found in fatty fish like salmon (as well as in fish oil capsules)—along with berries, beans, and greens. Compounds in berries fuel the body's cell-protecting antioxidant defenses. And the B vitamins in beans and greens support swift information processing inside your noggin.

LOOK
YOUNGER

DO YOU EAT RIGHT, EXERCISE FREQUENTLY, AND KEEP YOUR SMILE BRIGHT AND WHITE? Maybe you also impress people as smart, practical, and calm when things get tough. That's a recipe for looking good that we can all aspire to. And there are other things you can do to get high marks on looking pretty darned attractive!

Wearing sunscreen *every time* you go outside could, quite quickly, help you look 24% younger than if you'd skipped it (more than 30% of Americans go without it). That's the impressive news from a 2013 study that tracked the sunscreen habits and microscopic facial wrinkles of 903 adults over four years.

Sunscreen use is one of many factors that can keep you looking younger than the rest of the world. Diets packed with fruit and vegetables feed a glowing, smooth complexion. And fitness habits can keep you trim, adding to your appeal.

In this chapter, you'll discover smart, affordable ways to care for your skin, hair, and smile.

TEST HOW SMART
YOU ARE ABOUT BEATING THE CLOCK

The secret to looking great can't be found solely in lotions, serums, or repair creams. Good health—and smart personal care—are key. Think you know how it's done? Take the quiz, then get the 411 on looking your youngest in the pages ahead.

1 **Stopping oral contraceptives can have this unexpected downside:**

a. Faster wrinkling

b. Yellowing teeth

c. Thinning hair

2 **This humble food is so good at soothing dry, itchy skin—even eczema—that top dermatologists routinely recommend adding it to a warm bath:**

a. Olive oil

b. Buttermilk

c. Oatmeal

3 **True or false:** Antibacterial soaps are a reliable way to protect yourself from germs.

4 **Cut your risk for dry skin in winter by:**

a. Taking a short bath or shower with warm—not hot—water and a mild soap

b. Gently patting your body dry

c. Briskly toweling off to stimulate circulation

5 **Strawberries and pineapple help keep teeth whiter because they contain:**

a. Natural scrubbing agents

b. Natural bleaching compounds

c. Fiber that acts like dental floss

6 **Getting enough protein from lean meat, skinless poultry, and fish can help your skin look younger by:**

a. Providing the building blocks your body uses to make collagen, which keeps skin looking firm

b. Keeping you lean, so you don't develop jowls or a flabby neck

c. Reducing inflammation

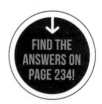

FIND THE ANSWERS ON PAGE 234!

REFORM

I was the poster child for sun damage when I was younger. I even skipped classes in college to tan! Then one day in my 30s, I caught a glimpse of myself in a mirror and thought, *Who's that old lady?* Now I apply moisturizer with SPF two to three times a day—yes, even in winter. I also have a bottle of fizzy mineral water every evening, which helps keep my skin hydrated overnight.

—NANCY SNYDERMAN, MD, FORMER CHIEF MEDICAL EDITOR, NBC NEWS

WHY IT WORKS → In addition to the impressive anti-aging research mentioned at the beginning of this chapter, in another landmark study, people who wore sunscreen regularly were 50% less likely to develop melanoma, the deadliest skin cancer, even though the study participants lived in Queensland, which has the highest rates of skin cancer in the world.

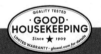

SUNSCREEN BUYING TIPS

GET RID OF ANY OPENED SUNSCREEN products from last season regardless of their expiration dates—it's highly likely that the protective ingredients have lost their potency from exposure to heat and the sun.

WHEN YOU'RE BUYING A NEW SUNSCREEN, look for one that's labeled broad-spectrum with a minimum of SPF 30. Broad-spectrum means protection from both UVA and UVB rays.

PRODUCTS WITH SPF VALUES HIGHER THAN 50 offer only minimal additional benefits, so don't be taken in by those high numbers.

CHECK PACKAGES FOR EXPIRATION DATES to make sure you're not buying old products.

—BIRNUR ARAL, PHD, DIRECTOR, GOOD HOUSEKEEPING HEALTH, BEAUTY AND ENVIRONMENTAL SCIENCES LAB

SKIP THIS INGREDIENT

I can be a fanatic about germs. As a physician, I know that most infections are spread by hand-to-mouth or hand-to-nose contact. So good hand washing is vital. But I avoid using antibacterial soaps that contain either triclosan or triclocarban, two similar bacteria-killing chemicals that may lead to antibiotic resistance. There's evidence that both can be harmful to health and the environment.

Triclosan interfered with muscle strength and heart function in an animal study at the University of California, Davis. In addition, it disrupted the activity of reproductive hormones and communication between brain cells. In male rats, triclosan also lowered sperm counts, damaged the reproductive system, and disrupted androgen production. The reason to worry about its effect on male rats is that male humans have identical hormones and hormone responses.

—GINA M. SOLOMON, MD, CLINICAL PROFESSOR OF MEDICINE AT THE UNIVERSITY OF CALIFORNIA, SAN FRANCISCO

WHY IT WORKS → Plain soap is really all you need. In fact, you won't even find triclosan and a host of similar antiseptic ingredients in soaps come the fall, thanks to a recent FDA ruling that established that over the counter hand and body washes containing them cannot be marketed after September 6, 2017. But triclosan is also often added to makeup, toothpaste, and all kinds of products labeled "antibacterial," including many cutting boards, yoga mats, towels, clothing, toys, and shoe liners. Does it help? Not much, with one exception. There's some evidence that adding triclosan to toothpaste reduces your risk of early gum disease (gingivitis). Otherwise, there's no proof of health benefits in any other products.

TAKE SKIN-FRIENDLY SHOWERS

It's tempting, especially in cold weather, to take long, hot showers. But they can be extremely drying to the skin. Keep baths and showers short and stick to warm water. Switching to an extra-mild cleanser in winter can help reduce itching and dryness. Afterward, gently pat your skin dry, don't briskly towel off—rubbing can be irritating.

—**STEPHEN P. STONE**, MD, FAAD, PROFESSOR OF DERMATOLOGY AND DIRECTOR OF CLINICAL RESEARCH, SOUTHERN ILLINOIS UNIVERSITY SCHOOL OF MEDICINE, SPRINGFIELD

 DRY SKIN IS WELL WORTH COMBATTING. IN A SURVEY OF 1,000 WOMEN:

✔ 20% said that flaky, parched skin interfered with sleep and sex, and sometimes even made them think twice about shaking hands

✔ 10% said it could put them in a bad mood

✔ 40% said it made them feel unattractive

✔ Over 20% said they'd give up dessert or morning coffee to get rid of it

WHY IT WORKS → "Dry skin is a problem for many people in winter, and the older you are, the more protection your skin needs," says Stone. "I like combination cleanser/moisturizers for the shower, followed by a moisturizing cream after you dry off. If you use hand sanitizers, buy the kind with built-in moisturizers."

More good ways to keep skin moisturized and feeling good: Avoid deodorant soaps and skin products containing alcohol or fragrances—all can be irritating. Use hand cream after every hand washing. After you brush your teeth at night, use hand cream again and smooth a little petroleum jelly on extra-dry areas to encourage overnight repair.

EAT RIGHT FOR DEEP-DOWN HEALTHY SKIN

These days, anti-aging cosmetics can seem more like food than beauty potions: Everything from pomegranate to soy is being infused into creams, cleansers, and serums. But applying products to your skin's surface is no substitute for eating foods that nurture it from within. "Nutrition plays an important part in limiting aging and helping to protect your looks from sun damage, the number one cause of lines and wrinkles," says Adam Friedman, MD, associate professor of dermatology and director of translational research at George Washington School of Medicine, Washington, DC.

Recent research has pinpointed specific nutrients that help prevent harm from environmental factors, hydrate your complexion, and keep skin cells functioning properly. These four anti-agers belong on your plate.

1 VITAMIN C–PACKED PRODUCE. In a British study of 4,015 women, those with higher intakes of vitamin C had fewer wrinkles and softer skin. It makes sense, because vitamin C is a powerful antioxidant that helps protect skin at the cellular level. "Antioxidants prevent damage to cells and DNA that can interfere with the production of collagen, the main support structure for your skin," explains Friedman.

WHAT TO EAT Aim for 75 milligrams of vitamin C a day from food. Translation: Eat a navel orange at breakfast and five strips of yellow pepper in a lunchtime salad. Or have a cup of broccoli with dinner and a bowl of strawberries for dessert. Other abundant, delicious sources of C: melons, grapefruits, red peppers, tomatoes, grapefruit, and kale.

Bonus: Beta-carotene—found in carrots, cantaloupe, apricots, orange squash, and sweet potatoes—may increase collagen production and help your skin stay moist.

2 LEAN PROTEIN. In the same British study, women with low protein intakes had a more wrinkled appearance. "Protein provides the building blocks of skin-supporting collagen," says F. William Danby, MD, clinical assistant professor at Geisel School of Medicine at Dartmouth.

WHAT TO EAT Skinless poultry, egg whites, and fish are top lean protein choices. But well-trimmed low-fat cuts of pork and beef, such as loin and round, are okay, too, as is tofu. In fact, one small Japanese study found that women who consumed tofu-like soy extract for 12 weeks had fewer fine lines around their eyes and greater elasticity in their skin.

3 AVOID SUGAR. Individuals with high sugar intakes show an aged, sallow appearance. "Sugar leads to glycation, making natural turnover and repair of collagen impossible," says Danby.

WHAT TO EAT Avoid sugar in any form whether added to coffee or tea, present in sugary sodas and candy, hidden in peanut butter, or produced by digestion of high glycemic index foods like white bread, potatoes, cakes, cookies, many cereals, and sweetened flavored nondairy milks.

4 FATTY FISH. Sea fare like salmon guards against aging sun damage by bringing a hefty dose of omega-3 fatty acids to the table. In addition to the many other benefits attributed to omega-3s throughout this book, three British studies show that these fatty acids fight sunburn, and there's some evidence that they may protect collagen and deter skin cancer.

WHAT TO EAT Aim for three servings a week of foods high in omega-3s. Besides salmon, good choices include mackerel, herring, sardines, and lake trout. If you're not partial to fish, go for walnuts, flaxseeds, canola oil, pumpkin seeds, and tofu. They contain a compound (ALA) that the body converts into omega-3s, though it takes a lot of ALA to get adequate amounts.

5 WHOLE GRAINS. When you replace refined white rice and white-flour breads, cakes, and pasta with whole grains, you almost immediately reap a benefit. "Refined grains can raise insulin levels, which cause inflammation that damages the skin," says Friedman. Whole grains are also a good source of selenium, which protects against sun injury and is linked with a nearly 60% reduction in nonmelanoma skin cancers.

WHAT TO EAT Grains rich in selenium include brown rice, oatmeal, barley, and whole wheat. Aim for three to five servings a day—a morning bowl of oatmeal and a sandwich on whole-wheat toast gets you three *servings without thinking about it.*

FIVE SKIN CANCER TIPS

Follow these rules to help prevent skin cancer, which is currently the most common cancer in the United States.

1 **DON'T SKIMP.** Slather sunscreen on cancer-prone spots like the tips of the ears, back of the neck, and tops of the feet—and everywhere else, too. Use an ounce or more (the amount in a shot glass) and repeat at least every two hours. "Studies show that the average person uses about a third of that and doesn't reapply nearly often enough," says Anthony Peterson, MD, assistant professor and director of dermatology at Loyola University Chicago.

2 **NO EXCEPTIONS.** Don't think you can skip sunscreen if you have dark skin. "Patients are always surprised when I tell them that Bob Marley died of skin cancer," says Brooke Jackson, MD, founder and medical director of Skin Wellness Dermatology Associates in Durham, North Carolina. Although deadly melanoma is more prevalent in Caucasians, African Americans have a much lower survival rate—probably due to later diagnosis and to higher rates of cancer in surprising places that don't get much sun exposure, such as feet, under fingernails and toenails, and at the groin, says Jackson. "When you go for a skin exam, remove nail polish," she suggests. "If you frequently have manicures, look at your nails when the polish is off."

3 **THINK BIG.** A big wide-brimmed hat that completely covers your face and neck is as crucial as sunscreen. "A baseball cap covers just the forehead and maybe a bit of nose, but that leaves your ears, neck, most of your face, and the rest of your nose exposed," says Peterson.

4 **HOG THE SHADE.** Especially between 10 a.m. and 2 p.m. That's when the sun's rays are strongest. If you're at an all-day picnic or double-header baseball game, reapply sunscreen every two hours. And consider sun-protective clothing with a high SPF. "I particularly like those surf shirts for kids that protect their shoulders and neck," says Peterson.

5 **FAKE, DON'T BAKE.** The *only* safe tan is the one you get from a bottle. Don't be fooled by those "safer than the sun" signs you see at some tanning salons, says Peterson. Even though tanning bed lamps emit primarily UVA radiation, not UVB, it also causes skin cancer. "Tanning beds are actually worse than the sun," says Peterson, "because you can go in for just 10 minutes and end up with a really bad burn."

FIGHT WRINKLES NATURALLY

Sure, we call them laugh lines and say they're signs of a life well-lived . . . still, wouldn't you rather skip the wrinkles? These two home treatments, recommended by skin experts, help keep skin smooth and you looking younger:

✔ **SNACK ON SUPERFOODS. Try these three line-softening nibbles:**

ALMONDS. They're packed with skin-plumping good fats and vitamin E, a powerful antioxidant that helps offset damage from the sun's UV rays.

DARK CHOCOLATE with a cacao content of 72% or higher. It's also rich in DNA-protecting, damage-defying antioxidants.

BLUEBERRIES. They provide a potent combo of anti-aging antioxidants and vitamin C, which helps protect collagen, the supportive protein that helps keep skin looking smooth and wrinkle-free.

 "Skin is a matrix of proteins, water, and fats that needs a healthy food supply for replenishment," says New York City dermatologist David Colbert, MD, author of *The High School Reunion Diet*. That goes for snacks, too.

✔ **MASSAGE AWAY STRESS. You can soothe and smooth tired, stressed-out skin with relaxing, do-it-yourself acupressure.**

Using your index and middle fingers, massage between your brows for 20 rotations.

Apply light pressure to temples for 10 seconds, then to your jawbone joint (located in front of your ears) for 10 seconds. Repeat.

Lightly press the muscle that protrudes when you clench your teeth for five to 10 seconds.

 These moves will release tension and, used regularly, may even increase skin elasticity a bit, according to Maya Kron, LAc, a licensed acupuncturist in the New York City area.

SKIN BARGAINS WORTH BUYING

Not interested in spending big bucks on scary injections or high-end beauty products with big price tags? Drugstore products often work just as well. "Much of the time, the biggest difference between a low-end and high-end product is the packaging, not the ingredients," says Debra J. Wattenberg, MD, assistant clinical professor of dermatology at Mount Sinai Medical School in New York City. Compare labels for the percentage of active ingredients that plain and fancy products contain (they're listed from most to least).

New York City dermatologist Debra Jaliman, MD, author of *Skin Rules*, suggests three types of treatment bargains that can erase the years.

1 **PRODUCTS CONTAINING RETINOL. Dark spots and uneven texture are instant agers. Keep fooling folks by applying a retinol treatment every night.**

WHY IT WORKS "Retinol is one of the few things that reverses sun damage," says Jaliman. "It will lighten brown spots, improve texture, and make skin smoother. You'll see a difference in weeks." Just be extra-sure to use at least an SPF 30 during the day because retinols make skin particularly sensitive to sunlight.

2 **MOISTURIZERS WITH CYTOKINES. Less well known than antioxidants but perhaps more effective, cytokines have been shown by medical studies to improve the appearance and texture of skin, reducing fine lines, wrinkles, and roughness. They're also unlikely to irritate skin, making them ideal for everyday use.**

WHY IT WORKS Cytokines, a naturally occurring plant growth factor, have been shown to stimulate cellular growth and collagen production.

3 **A SONIC CLEANSING BRUSH. Jaliman finds sonic cleansing devices (those handheld oscillating brushes, like Clarisonic) far more effective ways to exfoliate dry, dead cells—without irritating your skin—than run-of-the-mill facial scrubs. Drugstores now carry affordable versions of these cleansing devices.**

WHY IT WORKS "A lot of what makes people look older is a buildup of dry skin," says Jaliman. "I've actually used an exfoliant scrub and then used a white towel, and I see how much aging dead skin, not to mention makeup and dirt, is still on my face," she says. "You use a sonic cleansing system and you see there's nothing left."

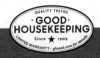

PROVEN ANTI-AGING ACTIVES
TO LOOK FOR IN SKIN CARE

HYALURONIC ACID. Naturally present in the human body, this substance is a super moisturizer. Also used in injectable fillers, it is found in many topical cosmetics formulated to plump and hydrate.

NIACINAMIDE. A water-soluble vitamin that is part of the vitamin B family, this ingredient is a multitasker. It has anti-inflammatory and skin-whitening properties, and it helps skin retain moisture by strengthening its outer layer. It also helps increase the production of collagen, a protein essential to keeping skin firm and smooth.

GLYCOLIC ACID. It's a key member of the alpha hydroxy acids, a group of chemical exfoliators that loosen the "glue" between dead cells, so they slough off to reveal fresh skin. It can be found in anti-aging products—peels, for example—that promise to reduce fine lines and even out skin tone.

PEPTIDES. These short-chain proteins/amino acids are involved in many biological processes, such as cell communication. Cosmetic companies have developed proprietary blends of peptides that target specific anti-aging processes in skin, like collagen production.

—**BIRNUR ARAL**, PHD, DIRECTOR, GOOD HOUSEKEEPING HEALTH, BEAUTY AND ENVIRONMENTAL SCIENCES LAB

10-SECOND SOLUTIONS

SIP SKIN-FRIENDLY GREEN TEA

Green tea is rich in polyphenols, antioxidants that are also anti-inflammatory and help sun-damaged skin cells repair themselves more efficiently. That could reduce your risk for nonmelanoma and melanoma skin cancer. That's not all. "Regularly drinking two to three cups a day will also improve skin texture and inhibit wrinkling," says Santosh K. Katiyar, PhD, professor of dermatology, University of Alabama at Birmingham.

SAY NO TO SPECIAL SKIN VITAMINS

"Nutricosmetic" pills (drinks, too) claim to deliver essential fatty acids, antioxidants, and other plant extracts linked in lab studies with reduced facial lines and wrinkles. But they're expensive and may or may not work. Simply eating four to five cups of fruits and vegetables provides even more of the vitamins, minerals, and other nutrients that enhance skin—and these healthy foods help your body in many other ways, according to Diane L. McKay, PhD, of the Friedman School of Nutrition Science and Policy at Tufts University, Boston.

SHUN AGING FAT

Another reason to avoid artery-clogging saturated fat: Beyond its role in promoting heart disease, sat fat—the type found in marbled meats and full-fat dairy products—may also make you look older. "Eating a lot of saturated fat induces skin-aging inflammation," says Jane Grant-Kels, MD, founding chair emeritus of the dermatology department at the University of Connecticut in Farmington.

SURPRISING FIXES FOR SKIN AND NAIL TROUBLES

Warts? Nail fungus? Dry, scaly skin? Reach into your toolbox, your kitchen cabinet, and your collection of cold-care aids for these surprising do-it-yourself remedies.

DUCT TAPE TO REMOVE WARTS. It might help. In 2002, a group of doctors compared duct tape's effectiveness with liquid nitrogen in removing warts. After two months of wearing duct tape on a daily basis and using a pumice stone about once a week to exfoliate the dead skin, 85% of patients' warts were gone, whereas freezing removed only 60%.

WHY IT MIGHT WORK "The question is whether there is something in the chemical adhesive itself, or if the occlusion (suffocation) causes the destruction of the wart," says Robin Blum, MD, a dermatologist in New York City. "The other thinking is that the duct tape causes irritation, which stimulates our body's immune cells to attack the wart."

VAPOR RUB TO CURE NAIL FUNGUS. Unlike duct tape, this popular remedy has yet to be tested, but doctors have heard plenty of success stories from patients who say regularly slathering a fungus-riddled toenail with vapor rub eventually knocks out the problem.

WHY IT MIGHT WORK "Many people swear it helps. I'm just not sure why," Blum says. Some believe it's the menthol in the balm that kills the fungus; others say it's the smothering effect of the thick gel. Regardless, used consistently, somehow vapor rub gets rid of not just the fungus but also the infected toenail, which turns black and eventually falls off. When a new nail grows in, expect it to be fungus-free.

OATMEAL TO SOOTHE ECZEMA. "Oats have anti-inflammatory properties," Blum explains. Most skin experts recommend treating rough, inflamed, itchy skin areas with wet colloidal (finely ground) oatmeal for at least 15 minutes, whether it's used as a paste or poured into a bath.

WHY IT MIGHT WORK In addition to reducing inflammation, oats are believed to have an antihistamine effect. By reducing histamine, which triggers inflammation, Blum explains, oats reduce eczema's redness.

MEN'S SKIN NEEDS TLC, TOO

While men's skin is tougher and thicker than women's, it's actually often more sensitive. Men's skin loses moisture faster, is more prone to dryness, and doesn't naturally exfoliate as well. But you can't give most men a multi-step skin-care regimen because they simply won't do it.

Instead, try one thing at a time that's a clear problem solver. For instance, my husband now loves an alcohol-free toner that contains calendula, which soothes his skin. He finds that using it after shaving counteracts any irritation.

Some men need extra anti-acne care, especially if they work out or play sports regularly. Sweating clogs pores. If they have oily skin and are prone to breakouts, they'll have fewer problems if they use a cleanser with glycolic or salicylic acid on their face. The acids exfoliate and balance the skin.

Guys with very oily skin should consider a gel that combines benzoyl peroxide with oil-absorbing ingredients. If they break out on their chest, back, or shoulders, cleansing products with benzoyl peroxide will unclog these areas.

—NATALIE SEMCHYSHYN, MD, ASSISTANT PROFESSOR, DEPARTMENT OF DERMATOLOGY, DIVISION OF COSMETIC AND LASER SURGERY AT SAINT LOUIS UNIVERSITY SCHOOL OF MEDICINE

WHY IT WORKS → Semchyshyn adds, "men should use a gentle cleanser that doesn't strip away natural skin oils and aggravate dryness. They should try a moisturizer afterward, too. An all-in-one product that combines moisturizer, antioxidants, and sunscreen is an even better way to go." Look for unfussy, man-friendly moisturizers with familiar skin protectors such as vitamins C and E, as well as newer therapeutic ingredients, such as phloretin (an antioxidant derived from apples) and ferulic acid (another plant antioxidant). Both protect skin from the sun's UV rays, which speed wrinkling and up skin cancer risk.

THINNING HAIR IN WOMEN

Most women know that stress can lead to hair loss, but they may not realize that hair can fall out three months after they stop taking oral contraceptives, due to a drop in estrogen levels. Talk to your doc about adjusting your hormones.

—**ELISE M. BRETT**, MD, ENDOCRINOLOGIST IN NEW YORK CITY AND ASSOCIATE CLINICAL PROFESSOR AT THE ICAHN SCHOOL OF MEDICINE, MOUNT SINAI HOSPITAL

 "If a hormonal issue is related to your hair thinning, taking estrogen can help but it can also heighten some women's risk of blood clots, so discuss this option thoroughly with your physician," says Brett. "Biotin supplements are a safer option—take five mcg daily. And switch to a sulfate-free shampoo, which is a lot easier on your hair." In addition, hair loss can be a sign of male hormone (androgen) excess. An endocrinologist can properly evaluate and treat these conditions.

FOODS THAT WHITEN TEETH

Most people know that coffee, tea, and red wine stain teeth. So can blueberries and tomato/barbecue sauces. That doesn't mean you have to swear off them! Just try to rinse your mouth with water right after eating. Or stash sugar-free gum in your pocket or purse and chew it post-meal to stimulate teeth-cleaning saliva.

Then consider adding foods and drinks that encourage whiter teeth, which include pineapple, cheese, strawberries, apples, and celery.

—**LISA R. YOUNG**, PHD, RD, CD, ADJUNCT PROFESSOR, DEPARTMENT OF NUTRITION, FOOD STUDIES, AND PUBLIC HEALTH AT NEW YORK UNIVERSITY AND AUTHOR OF *THE PORTION TELLER PLAN*

 "Pineapple is rich in bromelain, a stain-removing enzyme, so at a cocktail party, order up a vodka and pineapple juice. Cheese boosts the pH level in your mouth, which strengthens tooth enamel. Strawberries are chock-full of malic acid, a tooth-whitening agent, and crunchy fruits and veggies like apples and celery help scrub away stains as you chew.

ANSWERS TO
HOW SMART YOU ARE ABOUT BEATING THE CLOCK

1 **C.** The sudden drop in estrogen when a woman stops taking oral contraceptives can shut down some hair follicles. After a few months, hair seems thinner, but because of the time delay, the connection isn't obvious so you may have a tough time figuring out the cause. One way to encourage hair growth is by taking a biotin supplement. *See page 233.*

2 **C.** Adding oats to your tub can reduce inflammation and be a major balm for dry, red, itchy skin and skin bothered by eczema. Finely ground "colloidal" oats, designed for use in the bath, are best, but dry oats from the kitchen will do in a pinch. *See page 231.*

3 **FALSE.** According to the FDA, triclosan—one of the most common antibacterial compounds in germ-fighting soaps—has no health benefits, with one possible exception: used in toothpaste, it may reduce risk for early gum disease. Otherwise, it's not only ineffective but may threaten both human fertility and the environment. Top docs suggest washing your hands regularly with regular soap. *See page 222.*

4 **A AND B.** A long hot bath or shower can make you feel toasty on a winter night but also dry out your skin. Protect yours with brief baths or showers in warm water and an extra-mild soap. Pat dry and moisturize afterward. *See page 223.*

5 **B.** Your fruit salad could keep your teeth whiter if it includes strawberries and pineapples. Strawberries contain a tooth-whitening compound called malic acid and pineapple has bromelain, an enzyme that helps remove stains. Sweet! *See page 233.*

6 **A.** In one British study, women who skimped on protein had more wrinkles than those who got enough. Protein helps bolster collagen fibers, the skin's internal support system. Bonus: Getting protein from fish like salmon also provides omega-3 fatty acids, which help protect skin against sun aging and skin cancer. *See page 224.*

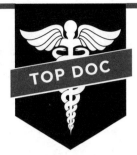

REMEMBER THESE FIVE STRATEGIES FOR LOOKING GREAT

Follow this natural regimen and you'll look forward to looking in the mirror. It pulls together top docs' most powerful "look great" advice and puts it into one simple plan.

1 **WEAR SUNSCREEN EVERY DAY.** You've read it elsewhere in this book and it bears repeating. Sunscreen is proven to cut risk for deadly skin cancers and to slow skin wrinkling. Start today and you'll look years younger in the future.

2 **EAT FOR HEALTHY SKIN.** The same menu that keeps the threats of heart disease and diabetes in check also feeds your skin. We're talking about fruit, vegetables, whole grains, lean meats, and fish. Sip a cup of green tea, too. Its polyphenols soothe reddening inflammation and even help sun-damaged cells repair themselves.

3 **BE OPEN TO OFFBEAT BUT DOC-RECOMMENDED REMEDIES.** Duct tape for warts. Oatmeal baths to soothe irritated skin. Vapor rub for toe fungus. Fruit for tooth whitening. Doctors aren't sure why some of them work, but work they do.

4 **THINK TWICE ABOUT ANTIBACTERIAL SOAPS.** It's wise to wash your hands to stop the spread of germs. But plain soap is all you need. Some common antibacterial ingredients used in soap and many other products are causing disturbing health problems in lab studies—while delivering almost no health benefit. Pass them by.

5 **GUYS: BABY YOUR SKIN, TOO.** Skin care isn't just for women and little ones. Men who care about their skin's looks and health should pay attention to preventing sun aging and skin cancer, controlling acne, keeping skin moisturized, and soothing irritation from shaving. Put your best face forward.

INDEX

Note: Page numbers in *italics*/parentheses indicate answers to tests

HEARSTBOOKS

An Imprint of Sterling Publishing Co., Inc.
1166 Avenue of the Americas
New York, NY 10036

GOOD HOUSEKEEPING is a registered trademark
of Hearst Communications, Inc.

This publication is intended for informational purposes only. The publisher
does not claim that this publication shall provide or guarantee any benefits, healing,
cure, or any results in any respect. This publication is not intended to provide or replace
conventional medical advice, treatment, or diagnosis or be a substitute to consulting
with a physician or other licensed medical or health-care provider. The publisher shall
not be liable or responsible in any respect for any use or application of any content
contained in this publication or any adverse effects, consequence, loss, or damage
of any type resulting or arising from, directly or indirectly, the use or application of
any content contained in this publication.

Any trademarks are the property of their respective owners, are used for editorial
purposes only, and the publisher makes no claim of ownership and shall acquire
no right, title, or interest in such trademarks by virtue of this publication.

ISBN 978-1-61837-226-0

Distributed in Canada by Sterling Publishing Co., Inc.
c/o Canadian Manda Group, 664 Annette Street
Toronto, Ontario, Canada M6S 2C8
Distributed in Australia by NewSouth Books
45 Beach Street, Coogee, NSW 2034, Australia

For information about custom editions, special sales, and premium
and corporate purchases, please contact Sterling Special Sales
at 800-805-5489 or specialsales@sterlingpublishing.com.

Manufactured in the United States of America.

2 4 6 8 10 9 7 5 3 1

www.sterlingpublishing.com

Design by Nancy Leonard

Cover: © Valentina Razumova/Shutterstock. Icons: Depositphotos, iStock.